I0049957

SFIMMS SERIES IN NEUROMUSCULOSKELETAL MEDICINE

FUNCTIONAL METHODS
IN OSTEOPATHIC
MANIPULATIVE MEDICINE

Non-allopathic Approaches to the Assessment and Treatment of Disturbances in the Mechanical Relations of the Neuromusculoskeletal System

HARRY D. FRIEDMAN DO FAAO

FUNCTIONAL METHODS
IN OSTEOPATHIC
MANIPULATIVE MEDICINE

Non-allopathic Approaches to the Assessment and Treatment
of Disturbances in the Mechanical Relations of the
Neuromusculoskeletal System

HARRY D. FRIEDMAN DO FAAO

Assistant Clinical Professor

Department of Family Medicine, College of Osteopathic Medicine
Michigan State University
East Lansing, Michigan

Touro University College, Vallejo, CA

Western University
College of Osteopathic Medicine, Pomona CA

New York College of Osteopathic Medicine
Old Westbury, NY

Illustrations David M. Driscoll DO

FUNCTIONAL METHODS
IN OSTEOPATHIC
MANIPULATIVE MEDICINE

Non-allopathic Approaches to the Assessment and Treatment
of Disturbances in the Mechanical Relations of the
Neuromusculoskeletal System

Copyright 2017 by Harry D. Friedman, first edition

All rights reserved. No part of this publication may be reproduced, stored
or transmitted in any form without prior authorization of the author and/
or illustrator

SFIMMS Press, Santa Cruz, California
www.sfimms.com
Library of Congress Control Number: 2017904479
ISBN: 978-0-9701841-6-0

Dedicated to

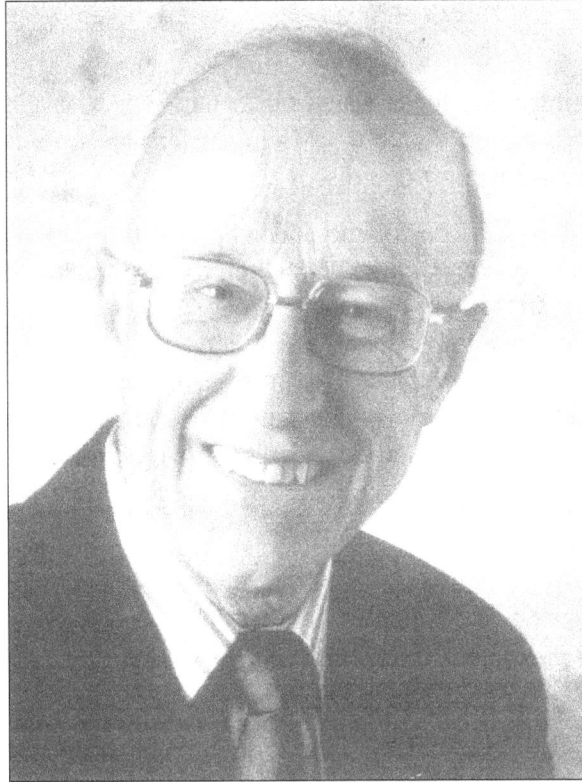

William L. Johnston DO FAAO
Developer of Functional Methods

February 17, 1921 -June 10, 2003

Like summer rain, you fell
with the gentle velocity of love
into my filled to capacity boat.

Capsizing, I swam
towards the distant wondrous shore
and you, like a perfect wave
lifted me effortlessly
bringing me breathlessly near
that sacred healing place.

But now I value even more
the thrill of the greatest ride
I shared with you!

FOREWORD TO THE EDITION

I arrived in East Lansing in the fall of 1983 to attend Osteopathic medical school. Being from California, my first impression of Michigan was, well,… flat…very flat. Fee Hall, home to the College of Osteopathic Medicine, rose high above the Michigan landscape, but was itself dwarfed by the "Osteopathic giants" inside, as I would soon discover.

I really had no idea what was in store for me and what transformation was about to occur in my perception of the world, in my very ability to perceive… Michigan State University College of Osteopathic Medicine (MSU-COM) was my school of choice mostly because of the fact that it boasted no less than 7 Fellow's of the American Academy of Osteopathy (FAAO's) in residence. Unfortunately, I soon found out that most of them were involved in research, administrative duties and patient care and didn't teach any formal classes to the students at all. So after recovering from this unbelievable disappointment, a few of my classmates and I decided to seek out the "Osteopathic giants" of Fee Hall.

What we experienced turned our lives upside-down and inside-out. How deceptive was the flatness of that place. Of course there were many notable "Osteopathic giants" that towered above the confines of Fee Hall, each of them revealing a different facet of Osteopathy that changed us, and our professional lives, forever. The true meaning of education, to bring forth, was never so clear as in those days of continuous mentoring with the remarkable faculty of MSU-COM.

I remember my first meeting with Bill Johnston. He was wearing a beige shirt, green plaid pants and a western bolo tie. His gentle demeanor and joyful countenance belied the intellectual bluntness of his ensuing discourse. He asked if I could tell him how an airplane stays its course. Being a student of systems theory and cybernetic principles, I informed him this was by way of the feedback of information about the plane's direction into the steering system's control mechanism. The actual direction of the plane was compared to the programmed direction and adjustments made which would steer the plane towards its set course.

He replied, "yes, and that's exactly how physiologic systems function as well, using feedback from sensory receptors to stay the course of the many biologic processes necessary for life." "So", he continued, "if the system can recognize that the airplane is off course and input the correct discrepancy to the control mechanism, then it will recalibrate itself to its original set-point and be back on course…. That is how the application of Functional Methods allows us to assess and treat disturbances within the motor control system." He explained, "the system has been designed to function symmetrically in reference to its midline. If the system moves asymmetrically and its midline has become disturbed, the clinician can introduce motor feedback which allows the system to re-establish its midline and recover its functional symmetry."

Dr. Johnston proceeded to demonstrate how he could palpate these discrepancies as asymmetries in the motion behavior of the motor system. With one hand he felt tension responses in the disturbed tissues as they attempted to comply with a simple motion demand (i.e. rotation) introduced by his other hand. Excessive responses were therapeutically countered with motion demands that reduced the tension response, providing sensory feedback that allowed the system to recognize the tension discrepancy (between disturbed and physiologic motion responses) and thereby re-establish symmetrical responses.

Dr. Johnston observed that though many tests could be applied to these areas of tissue disturbance, some tests were more reliable than others. One of Dr. Johnston's lifelong inquiries was developing reliable and reproducible tests for just this purpose. This uniformity of testing procedures was important to his way of thinking and applied to his teaching and research activities, as well as to clinical record keeping. It was his assertion that most of the tests used by the profession were not uniform or reliable and his research efforts were directed at validating basic testing procedures. Dr. Johnston authored and published more clinical studies on palpation and testing procedures than anyone in the Osteopathic profession. From knowledge gained through this research and through clinical observation, Dr. Johnston designed courses for developing clinical problem solving approaches to assess and treat these disturbed motion responses, focusing on palpation skills and uniform testing procedures.

Few could match the thoughtful rigor with which Dr. Johnston embraced Osteopathy; likewise, few could match the skill with which he applied it. He had a knack for finding key dysfunctions, usually in the ribcage, which would bring about a complete reorganization of the musculoskeletal system when resolved. As disciplined in his palpation as he was in his thinking, Bill left no stone unturned, checking for relationships between all body regions that might reveal a disturbance of clinical significance.

Osteopathic physician, Osteopathic educator, Osteopathic researcher, Bill Johnston, DO, FAAO excelled at each and aspired to them all in his unique blend of Osteopathy. But Bill Johnston was more than any of these things to me, and I think even he considered, or at least hoped, himself to be something more. To me, Bill was a revolutionary, a critical thinker and philosopher, with a hand on Osteopathic history and an eye on its evolution. He worked tirelessly to forward his revolution, in practice, in teaching and in research.

Dr. Johnston was a quiet rebel, he didn't draw attention to himself and never criticized those who didn't appreciate or understand his life's work. His revolution was a solo effort, as he had no army or faction to support his cause, nor was he out to recruit anyone and considered no one his enemy. Bill Johnston just went about his work, like a busy spider, weaving an intricate and delicate web of knowledge based on observation and confirmed through research. Some, like me, became ensnared in his web, caught by the originality and clarity of his ideas and observations. That's where Dr. Johnston's quiet revolution was waged and won, in the hearts and minds of his students and admirers.

There were so many questions I had that he never had the time to answer. In retrospect, I think, maybe he didn't want to answer them. If Bill Johnston's quiet revolution were to ever have any impact, the answers had to come from others in whom the revolution had taken hold. Even more, I think in Dr. Johnston's own mind, it was the investigation, not the answers, that spun the web of his revolution; observations, not arguments, were the threads which held it together and made it stick.

I invite you into the amazing world of Dr. Johnston. In the pages that follow we will explore fundamental concepts (some to embrace and some to abandon) in the practice of Osteopathy. For each region we will cover in detail, the tests used to discern and the criteria for making the diagnosis of somatic (motor system) dysfunction. We will present learning modules for palpatory skills development to directly perceive motor system disturbances and to introduce therapeutic forces to resolve them… and we will come back again and again to the basic question that Bill asked, "What is theory and what is fact?"

To quote Dr. Johnston: "If we cannot perceive factually what we are dealing with clinically, we'll never be able to successfully understand what is really going on in a dysfunctional neuro-musculoskeletal system. Reportable facts must be subjected to confirmation and acceptable levels of reliability in order to fulfill the major criteria of experimental research – reproducibility."

So many Osteopathic dreams have been awakened by knowing Bill, and destiny has even transformed the dreamer, as if awakening in the dream, the dreamer and the knower, one…There are no words to express my gratitude to Bill, only actions.

Harry D. Friedman DO, FAAO
Santa Cruz, California

TABLE OF CONTENTS

Course Objectives

1. Develop palpatory examination skills, which describe tissue and motor behavior (not structural alignment) using a progressive application of functional tests to identify, localize, and characterize somatic dysfunction.

2. Explore some of the theoretical aspects of a functional approach, which considers the relationship of regional and segmental musculoskeletal findings to physiologic disturbances of central control mechanisms and total body (homeostatic) functions.

3. Develop functional manipulative techniques for each body region based on altered tissue compliance and mobile responses to passive motion testing.

* Functional Methods is designed as an instructional manual. It is a condensed version of the text Functional Methods by Johnston and Friedman published by the American Academy of Osteopathy. Some additional new content has been added to the introductory sections and the last section on extremities.

FUNCTIONAL METHODS OVERVIEW

Applies unique palpatory problem solving skills to interact with the whole person and their physiology in a dynamic way. Develops practitioner's ability to perceive moment to moment behavior of the NMSK system by palpating segmental responses to motion demands placed on the entire body, observing whole body relationships not merely the structure and function of a single segment. By appreciating disturbances in the relationship between different parts of the body the practitioner can leverage the force vectors present between body regions and resolve them. Its not just correcting a single dysfunctional segment but removing a disturbance in the coordinated function of 2 or more parts within the whole body.

When a force enters the body it does not only create a disturbance at the point of contact, but because the entire body responds to the impact, disturbances occur in other body regions and normal relationships between difference parts of the body are altered. The resulting faulty mechanics can be appreciated using the palpatory skills taught in the Functional Methods course. These faulty mechanics create changes in motor programing that over time lead to postural and movement disorders that can be treated by addressing the underlying disturbance in the relationship between body regions caused by the original injury.

Local segmental testing and treatment frequently does not identify or resolve the disturbance in the relationship between different body regions and therefore the disturbance persists and the local dysfunction treated returns. Ultimately, when the relationship between body regions is restored, the inherent physiologic mechanism reboots the default program in the CNS, proper motor programming is resumed and subsequently more easily maintained.

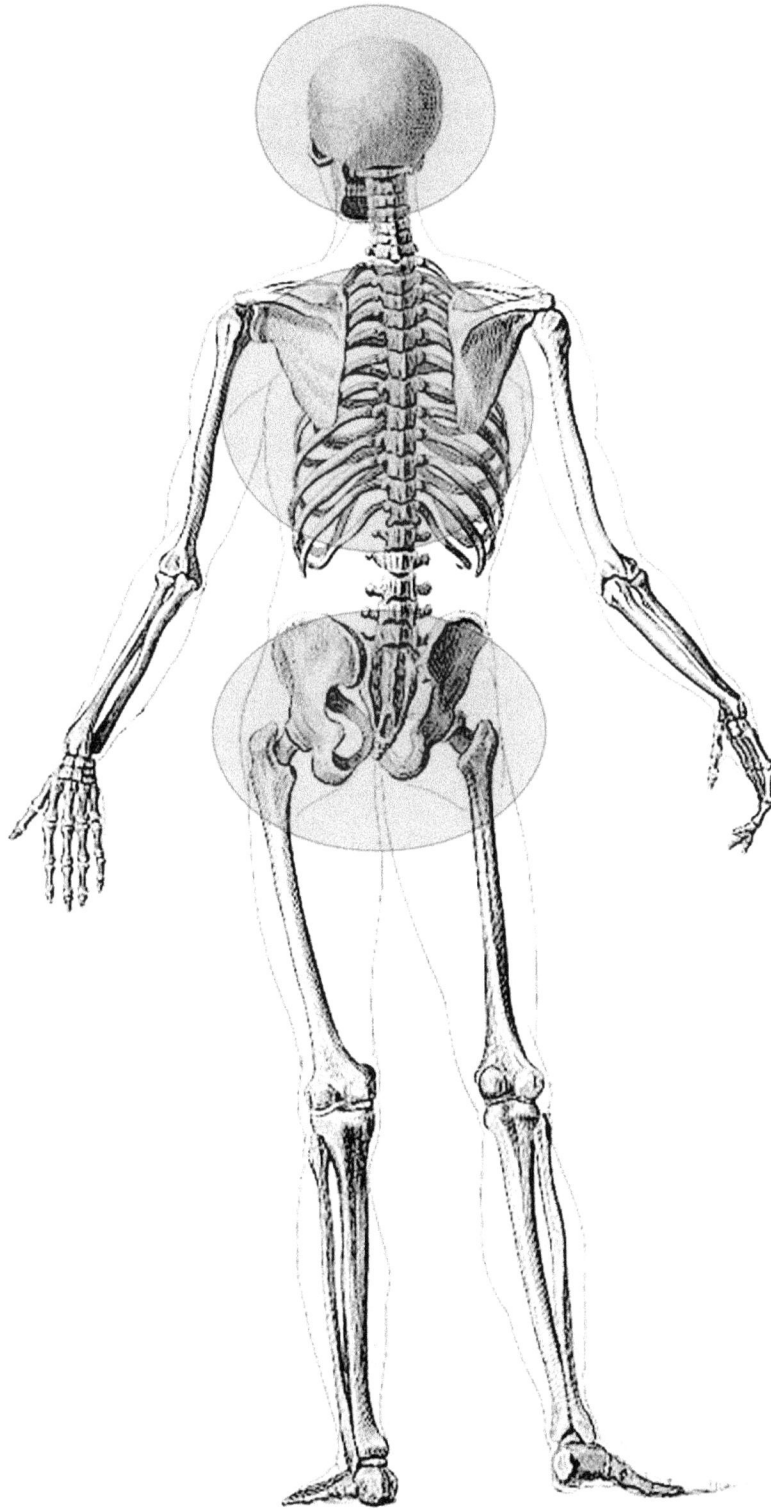

INTRODUCTION
to William L Johnston DO FAAO

William L. Johnston DO, FAAO, the primary developer of Function Methods, defined Osteopathic clinical research as "recorded observation of clinical findings and their response to treatment." His personal bias was that in the Osteopathic profession, more attention was placed on treatment methods than on the process used to elicit and describe palpable findings. He said "our thinking from the beginning has been our biggest impediment to progress." "In 100 years of clinical research and practice, the Osteopathic profession doesn't have a proper description of what it is we are treating". "The conceptual framework we have developed has limited our ability to observe what is actually going on."

He thought our focus on the idea of a joint fixation had programmed us to see and feel only this, when actually the joint is only one part of a larger motor feedback system. "What we expect to find has limited what we actually do find and even influences what we are able to feel by forcing us to interpret palpable findings in a manner consistent with our conceptual bias."

Dr. Johnston felt that in order to shift our thinking we must first make the distinction between fact and theory and in so doing realize that our perceptual apparatus has been altered by our cognition. Our ability to observe has been superceded by our fascination with theories and explanations. He said we needed to re-organize our thinking to focus on what is factual and retrain our palpation skills to perceive it.

In fact, the neuromusculoskeletal system is not a joint specific mechanism but rather a mobile system with mobile segments organized to meet and respond to the demands placed on the body as a whole...

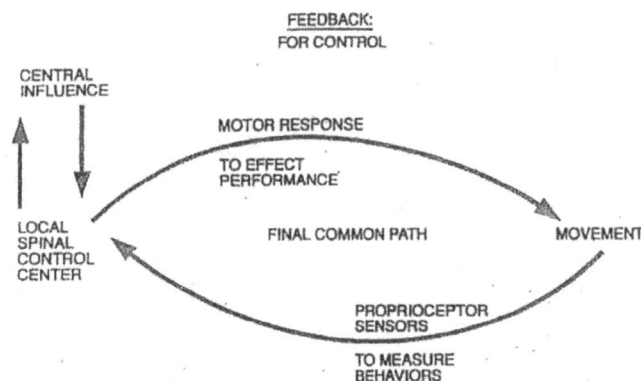

Motion (movement) is the organized output of the system and all the segments within that system follow the law of functional expression. "Tissues about a moving part constantly reflect mobile behavior as they comply with the demand for movement and positioning of the whole system." All the parts have to be in the right place at the right time to effect optimal behavioral performance. Position and structure are secondary aspects because they do not serve to describe primary behaviors within this dynamic functional system. "Position follows motion like a shadow. Motion is position on the run."

Dr. Johnston referred to the Dewey Doctrine and its utility for descriptive clinical research, "Observation, Dewey wrote, can become scientific if it is reported in direct relation to the particular procedure applied in the observance." Palpable findings can be factual observations when: 1. Tests used to elicit findings are described and reproducible 2. Criteria are clearly established for determining positive findings and 3. Description of finding is made in terms of the test used to elicit it

We will be describing specific tests with specific functional criteria to be applied to regional motor performance and to segmental behavior. Somatic dysfunction will be described in two ways. Regional somatic dysfunction reflects positive findings from the screening exam without regard for any segmental behavior. Segmental somatic dysfunction reflects tests which specifically focus on the exact location and character of disturbances which can be treated. Resolution of segmental somatic dysfunction should be accompanied by changes in regional performance as well.

Dr. Johnston· said, "If we cannot record factually what we are dealing with clinically then we will never be able to successfully explore what's really going on in a dysfunctional neuromusculoskeltal system." "Reportable facts must be subjected to confirmation, re-testing and acceptable levels of reliability in order to fulfill the major criteria for experimental research reproducibility!"

The Screening Exam

• The screening exam should afford a quick initial impression of gross problem areas and their relation to whole-body function and the overall health of the patient. Tests applied in a screening-level exam include regional motor asymmetry, regional structural asymmetry, and regional tissue quality.

• Screening tests are applied to all major body regions regardless of the location of pain or the patient's chief complaint, and without regard for segmental localization of findings.

• The screening exam then functions as a database for measuring basic functional parameters of the musculoskeletal system before, during, and after treatment interventions.

• Musculoskeletal examination employs visual and palpatory tests to locate and characterize areas of clinically relevant dysfunction.

> • Visual interpretation of structural relations evaluates deviation from the midline in three planes: coronal, sagittal, and transverse. Deviation from the midline can be observed in static posture as well as in dynamic posture (gait).

> • Palpatory perceptions reflect a dynamic interaction between the patient's tissues and the palpator's hand, which provides sensory information defined by detection, internal amplification, and interpretation. Palpatory interpretations include changes in:

temperature	tension
texture	thickness
surface humidity	shape
elasticity	irritability
turgor	motion

> • The screening exam should also assess the inherent vitality and overall health of the patient through both visual and palpatory means.

• Reproducibility of screening exam findings is dependent, then, on a standardized testing procedure as well as a record format that specifies which test was performed and whether the test was positive or negative. Reproducibility of the tests requires a common description of findings based on criteria for positive and negative responses.

• Standardization of the exam and its record may be useful for (1) communication between caregivers, (2) verifying diagnostic impressions, (3) monitoring outcome responses, (4) single- as well as multi-site data collection, (5) establishing educational standards, and (6) establishing practice standards.

SCREENING TESTS TO CHARACTERIZE
REGIONAL SOMATIC DYSFUNCTION

	ALTERED					
	Tiss Tex		Motion		Structure	
Head/face	27	28	47	48	12	13
Cervical	25	26	41	42	1	14
Thoracic	23	24	39	40	3	15
Lumbar	21	22	36	37	8	16
Sacro-pelvic	19	20	34	35	5	10
Costal Cage	31	32	44	45	2	9
Upper Extrem	29	30	38	46	4	11
Lower Extrem	17	18	33	43	6	7

STANDING STRUCTURE

❖ landmarks listing low to left or right?
  1 inferior mastoid process
  2 first rib (anterior to trapezius border)
  3 acromion
  4 inferior scapula
  5 superior iliac crest
  6 trochanter
  7 plantar arch

❖ 8 lumbar scoliotic curve? (convexity left or right)
  9 associated costal cage rotation? (left or right)

❖ anterior/posterior asymmetry (compare left and right)
  10 pelvis
  11 shoulders
  12 orbits

❖ 13 Does jaw deviate when relaxed and open? (left or right)

❖ A/P curves increased, decreased or normal?
  14 cervical
  15 thoracic
  16 lumbar

❖ Standardized for six tests per region:
   two tissue, two motion, two structure

❖ **Criteria for regional somatic dysfunction:**
   one positive tissue test **and**
   one positive motion **or** structure test
   in any one region

TISSUE

❖ Is there asymmetry of tissue tension laterally in:
  lower extremity: 17 calf?   18 thigh?
  19 gluteal?

❖ Is there a regional increase in paraspinal tissue tension that is larger than two spinal segments in:
  20 pelvis
  lumbar: 21 upper?   22 lower?
  thoracic: 23 upper?   24 lower?
  cervical: 25 upper?   26 lower?

❖ Is there asymmetry of tissue tension laterally in:
  jaw (masseter ms.):   27 relaxed?   28 clenched?
  upper extremity: 29 forearm?   30 upper arm?
  thoracic cage: 31 upper anterior? 32 lower lateral?

MOTION

❖ Is resistance encountered to introduction of passive:
  33 hyperextension at the knees? (compare left with right)
  34 lateral translation at the pelvis? (compare translation left with translation right)

❖ 35 Is posterior rotation of innominate bone restricted at PSIS with active unilateral
   hip flexion? (compare left with right)

❖ During active trunk sidebending:
  36 does the lumbar spine resist sidebending? (compare left with right)
     37 does rotation occur into the concavity? (non-neutral mechanics)

SEATED

❖ Is resistance encountered to introduction of passive:
  38 forearm pronation? (compare left with right)
  39 shoulder/trunk sidebending? (compare left with right)
  40 shoulder/trunk axial rotation? (compare left with right)
  41 head/neck sidebending? (compare left with right)
  42 head/neck axial rotation?(compare left with right)
  43 legs swing laterally? (compare left with right)

SUPINE

❖ During active inhalation, is resistance palpated in the thoracic cage:
  44 upper anterior? (compare left with right)
  45 lower lateral? (compare left with right)

❖ Is resistance encountered to introduction of passive:
  46 arms overhead? (compare left with right)

❖ Using the vault hold to assess cranial rhythmic impulse:
  47 Does vitality feel normal (strong), hyperactive or weak?
  48 Are flexion or extension restricted?

REGIONAL EXAM: MUSCULOSKELETAL SYSTEM

Required: The essential record of a screen for dysfunction during physical exam is formatted in the upper left table.

	ALTERED			Somatic Dysfunction
	Tissue Texture	Motion	Structure	
Head/face				
Cervical				
Thoracic				
Lumbar				
Sacro-pelvic				
Costal Cage				
Upper Extrem				
Lower Extrem				

Patient #: _____ M F

Date: _____ Age: _____

Comments: _____
_____
_____
_____
_____
_____
_____
_____

⊕ Presence of altered findings
⊖ Absence of altered findings
◎ Omitted

Somatic dysfunction = altered tissue texture + altered motion or structure

Make use of the Comments section above and the Diagrams below to facilitate description of the dysfuction when indicated:

Tissue: Circle the ⊗ for an area of increased tissue tension

Structure: Circle to indicate presence or absence of altered structural relations

Motion: Insert a barrier | for the direction of the restricted motion; circle appropriate letters

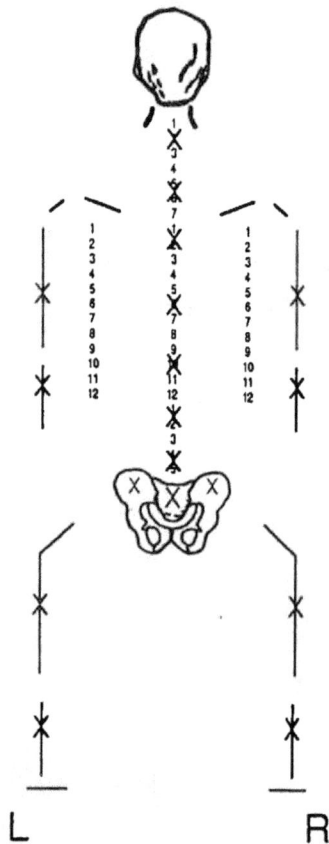

	L	R	=
Mastoid low	L	R	=
1st Rib low	L	R	=
Acromion low	L	R	=
Inf. Scapula low	L	R	=
Iliac Crest low	L	R	=
Trochanter low	L	R	=
Plantar Arch low	L	R	=
Lumbar Convexity	L	R	=
Costal Rotation	L	R	=
Pelvis anterior	L	R	=
Shoulder anterior	L	R	=
Orbit anterior	L	R	=
Jaw Deviated	L	R	=
Cervical Lordosis	↑	↓	N
Thoracic Kyphosis	↑	↓	N
Lumbar Lordosis	↑	↓	N

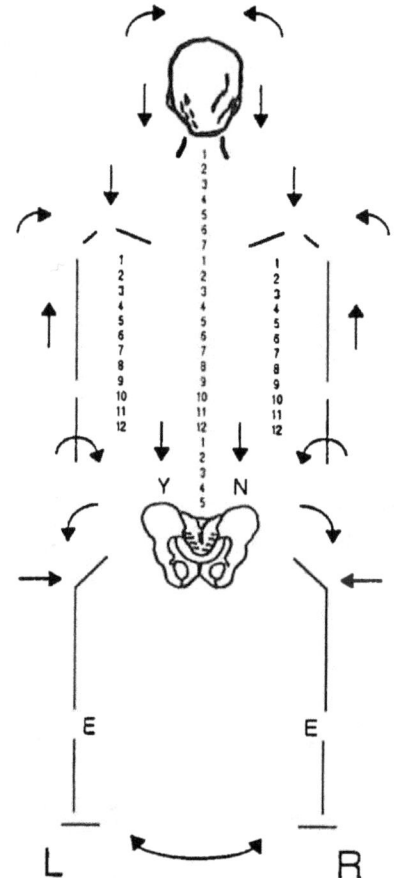

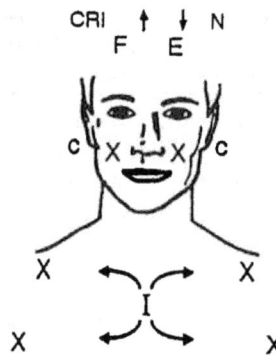

CRI ↑ ↓ N
F E

SIGNATURE

Scanning Procedures

Scanning tests help to localize the segmental locations of clinically significant areas of dysfunction. Scanning tests typically employ a repetitive, uniform test to elicit altered tissue behavior at a single segment. These behaviors include alterations of tissue texture, tissue tension, or tissue mobility. Segmental responses above and below area of dysfunction are typically opposite that of the central segment. Careful observation of responses to a single scanning test can help to localize dysfunction to a single central segment. Typical scanning procedures include:

- skin surface
- subcutaneous tension, texture tenderness
- passive gross motion
- active motion (inhalation)
- percussion

Percussion Scan

Percussion test is carried out from segment to segment using firm finger tension and a supple wrist. This allows the operator's hand to contact the tissue firmly, assessing its resistance to initial pressure as well as allowing the wrist to easily rebound or bounce in response to the elasticity of the muscle fibers. Increase in tissue resistance = decrease in tissue mobility. Decrease in rebound = increase in muscle tone.

Areas of maximal dysfunction that are characterized by performing the percussion test can be more closely examined by performing a deep shear or probe to assess the bogginess (or ropiness) of the deep subcutaneous tissues. (Bogginess = acute, ropiness = chronic.)

Respiratory Motion Scan

Mechanical functions of respiratory elements include anterior/posterior and lateral capacity of the thoracic cage to respond to motion demands of inhalation and exhalation (pump handle, bucket handle motions). The initial exhalation movement is passive, the active component of exhalation coming in the middle of the exhalation phase in order to control a smooth endpoint as the diaphragm relaxes and gravity accelerates. Diaphragm effort during inhalation is more immediate.

Breathing effort usually keeps the thoracic elements within an easy neutral phase of motion without developing tension in either the inhalation or exhalation direction. With dysfunction, this ease of movement is lost and tension increases reflecting an increased effort response to breathing locally. When we think of inhalation and exhalation as a demand for movement, then we expect mobile parts of the body to respond to breathing like any other motion, i.e., side-bending. Respiratory motion testing carried out repetitively at multiple segments in any part of the body, identifies areas of compliance or resistance.

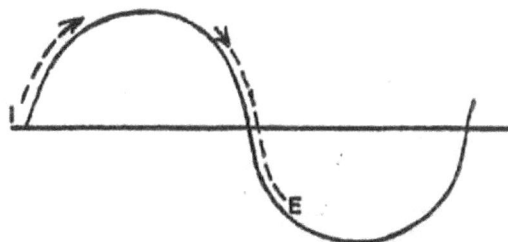

Scanning Exam Exercise

• Standing evaluation of thoracic and lumbar segments using percussion. Areas of maximal resistance are marked with the tape.

• Seated respiratory motion evaluation of thoracic areas identified using percussion scan. Test areas above and below with inhalation to begin mapping out a three-segment complex with opposite responses above and below the central segment.

• Use exhalation to observe opposite responses and to confirm the location of the central segment.

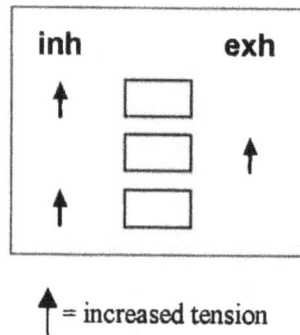

```
inh          exh
  ↑    ▭
       ▭     ↑
  ↑    ▭
```

↑ = increased tension

Side-Bending Motion Scan Exercise

• On a new partner, locate a central segment with an inhalation scan, confirming with the exhalation scan and additionally with side-bending of the thorax to the left and right.
• Side-bending responses should be noted as either increasing or decreasing in tension, comparing the response above and below the central segment to confirm the three segment complex.

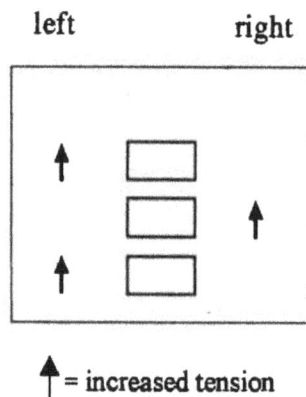

```
left          right

  ↑    ▭
       ▭     ↑
  ↑    ▭
```

↑ = increased tension

Segmental Motion Dysfunction

"Tissues about a moving bony part constantly reflect mobile behavior as they comply with demands for movement and positioning of the whole system."

Charles Bowles

Principles of a Functional Approach

- Functional principles focus on a data-gathering system that identifies actual behavior (motor responses). The students of this approach must set aside conceptual models which predict motion based on facet behaviors and structural relations.

- Motion testing is passive, and is carried out by introducing physiologic regional motions, not by testing a segmental response directly (i.e., pushing on the spinous process left or right). The motion response palpated is not positional, but dynamic, and not limited to a joint phenomenon.

- Mobile responses reflect disturbances in the relationship between body regions not merely misalignment of a single segment.

- All of the tissues surrounding the vertebral body comprise a unit that actively and passively influences the unique response of this patient, which can only be palpated. General rules or laws of vertebral motion describe normal situations and do not normally apply in clinical situations where the motor system has become altered.

- Since the nervous system is organized segmentally, the right and left sides of a particular mobile column within the body respond as a whole. In the functional terminology, we do not refer to a dysfunction being located on the left or on the right, but rather as a response of the whole column to left- or right-sided motions introduced passively from the operator.

- This sense of dysfunction is palpated as an initial asymmetry in the compliance/noncompliance (ease/bind) of a segmental response to motion; it is not the range of motion or the endpoint of motion that we are assessing. See graphs 1 and 2.

Graph 1   **Normal Mobile Segment**

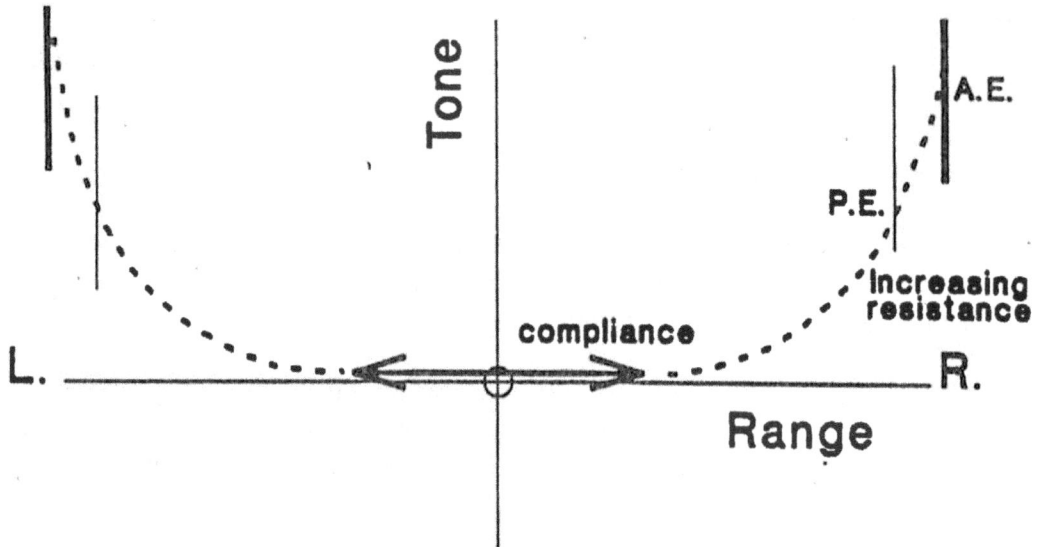

Graph 2   **Dysfunctional Mobile Segment**

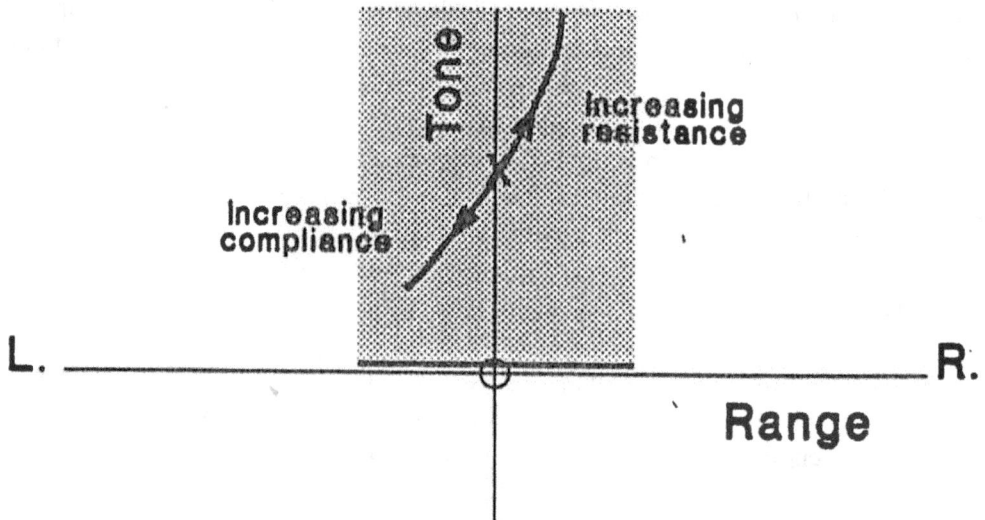

Functional Treatment Principles

- The palpating fingers of one hand become the listening hand, and they receive information from the deep tissues under the skin that are segmentally innervated. Motions are introduced by the other hand, the active hand, and incorporate rotary and translatory tests (three of each).

Rotary tests:	Translatory tests:
flexion/extension	anterior/posterior
side-bending left/right	lateral left/right
rotation left/right	axial distraction/compression

- Motion tests are introduced, and the operator assesses with the listening hand the responses of increasing and decreasing tension over an area of increased tissue tension assessed previously (i.e., percussion scan).

- Confirmation of segmental findings should be made by testing adjacent segments for mirror image (opposite) findings to the same motion demands. These adjacent levels above and below the central segment exhibit compensatory motion responses. Functional testing carried out at these adjacent segments helps to confirm the exact characteristics of the central segment. See Figure 1.

- Motor responses between these adjacent levels are perceived at the palpating fingers as relative difference of ease or bind. For example, a central segment that responds with an initial sense of tension to one motion is compared to the adjacent levels, which may exhibit considerably more tension. Compared to the adjacent levels, then, the central segment exhibits relative ease.

- Respiratory motion responses to inhalation and exhalation should also be tested and confirmed at adjacent levels.

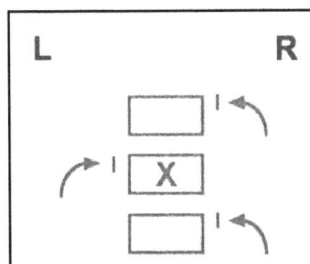

Figure 1.
Schematic representation of a fundamental unit of segmental dysfunction: A primary motor asymmetry is indicated at central segment X resisting rotation right, with compensatory opposing asymmetries at adjacent segments resisting rotation left.

Monitoring Segmental Responses

• Therapeutic motions can be applied to the central segment identified by either applying an indirect or direct principle. Consistent with the concept of afferent reduction, an indirect approach is primarily applied.

• Motions that produce a sense of ease or compliance in the listening hand are introduced and stacked one on the other until a sense of total tissue release occurs. All seven directions should be used, unless operator is not sure of motion response in one or more directions. The greater the number of directions, the better the response. This tissue release may be palpated as a sense of unwinding as the positioning changes slightly, moving into a greater sense of ease or compliance as the therapeutic response is achieved.

• Introduction of motions in each direction is small.

• Final step is introduction of respiratory motion, during which fine tuning of the other motions can occur.

• Retesting is essential. All findings should be completely resolved with symmetrical responses to motions introduced in both directions at all three segments.

• If two 3-segment complexes are in series (one right on top of the other) they may share one common segment which acts as the bottom segment for one and the top segment for the other 3-segment complex. In this case, after treatment, only 2 of the 3 segments will resolve, as the 3rd segment is still part of the remaining (untreated) 3-segment complex.

(Note: Rotation introduced in one region positions the adjacent region relatively rotated in the opposite direction. Head rotation left = trunk rotation right. Pelvic rotation right = trunk rotation left.)

Cervical Spine Treatment

- Seated deep tissue shear to locate areas of increased tissue tension

- Seated rotation scan to identify three-segment complex in an area of increased tissue tension.

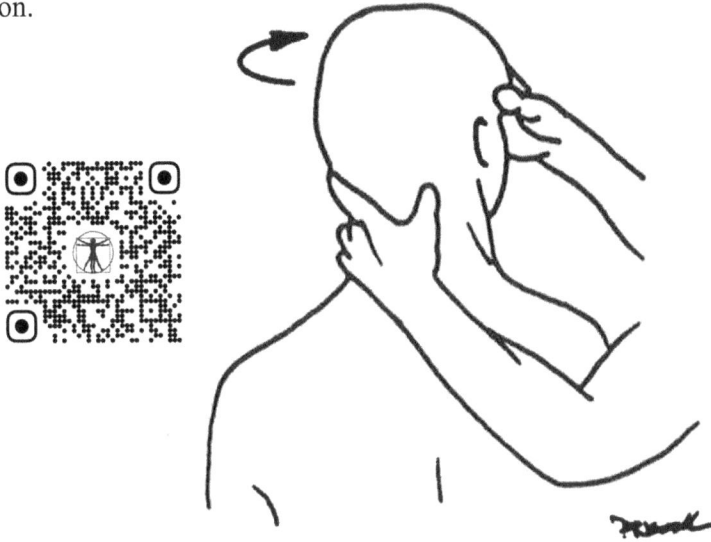

- Confirm in the seated position with inhalation and exhalation responses at all three segments.

- Supine treatment, operator sitting at head of table with elbows on knees to use as a fulcrum to introduce motions into the patient's head and neck.

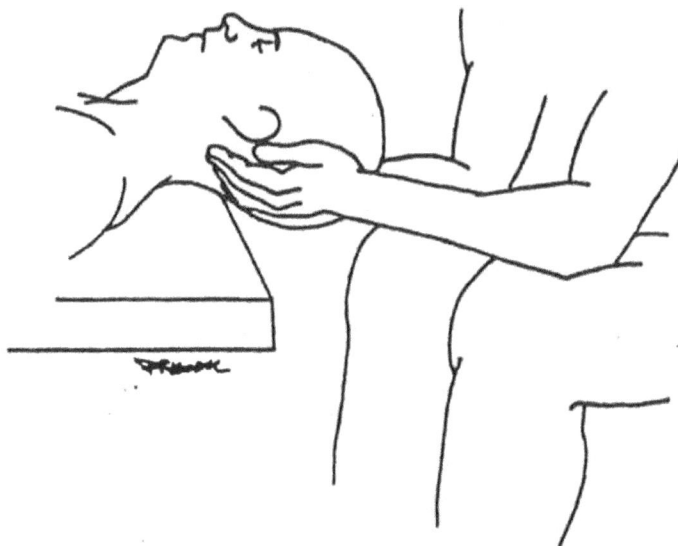

(A central segment at Cl has mirror images above at CO and below at C2. A central segment at CO has only a mirror image at Cl).

Thoracic Spine Treatment

- Seated percussion scan to locate areas of increased tissue tension.

- Seated rotation scan introducing motion through the patient's ipsilateral crossed arm.

- Three-segment complex is confirmed using inhalation and exhalation.

- Operator stands on the side of easy rotation at the central segment with their arm under the patient's to induce sidebending. The operator uses the patient's ipsilateral arm for side-bending in the opposite direction and contralateral arm for side-bending in the ipsilateral direction. Introduction of motion through head is effective for the thoracic segments T1-T5. Lower thoracic and upper lumbar segments can be treated supine using leg movements introduced from below.

- Additional mobile responses are tested and directions of ease added for flexion/extension, rotation right/left, anterior/posterior translation, translation left/right and compression/distraction. Extension may require the patient to sit lower, on a stool, and flexion may be assisted by having the patient sitting up higher, on a table.

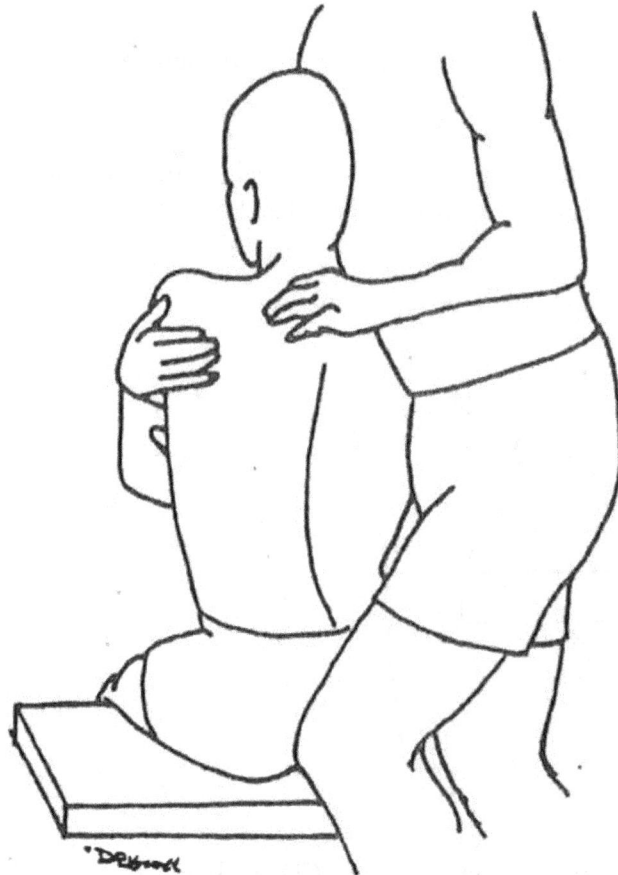

Functional Approach to the Thoracic Cage

• Thoracic cage dysfunctions occur in the left or right latral columns with mirror images occurring above and below the central segment. Additionally, for inhalation restrictions, mirror images can be found in the midline thoracic spine column as well. See Figure 8 & 9

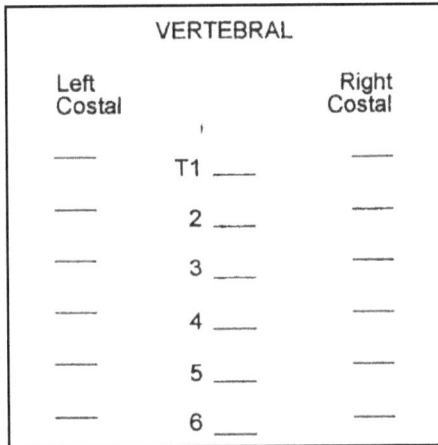

Figure 8. Schematic of central and lateral columns

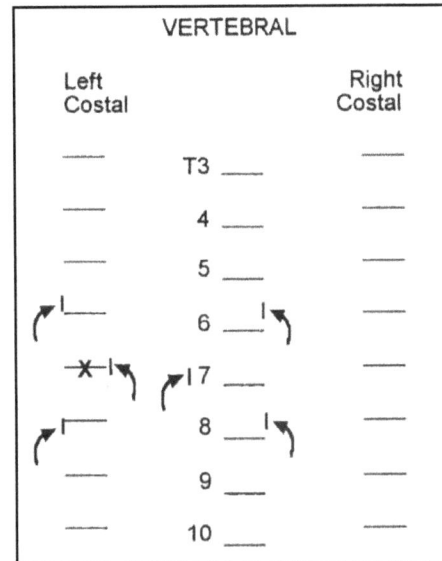

Figure 9. Schematic representation of primary dysfunction (X) at left rib 7 resisting active inhalation and passive rotation to the left. Secondary asymmetries are indicated at left ribs 6 and 8 within the left lateral vertical column.
Opposing vertebral asymmetries at T-6, T-7, and T-8 indicate a horizontal adaptation to the lateral costal dysfunction at left rib 7. (Arrows indicate directions of resistance to axial rotation tests only.)

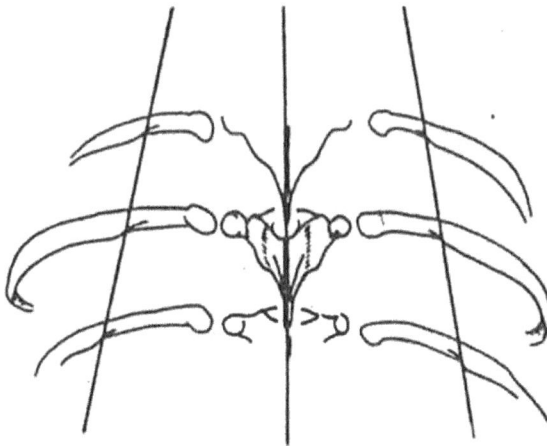

• Tissue and motion scans can be carried out supine or side-lying as well as seated using tissue resistance to pressure, rotation, and respiratory responses.

• Once the central segment has been confirmed, treatment can be carried out in the side lying position using the ipsilateral upper extremity to introduce motions responding with increasing ease at the dysfunctional central rib. (See Figure 10)

• Treatment continues with trunk positioning performed in the seated position to address the axial rotary and translatory motion responses at the dysfunctional rib. (See Figure 11)

Functional Approach to the Thoracic Cage

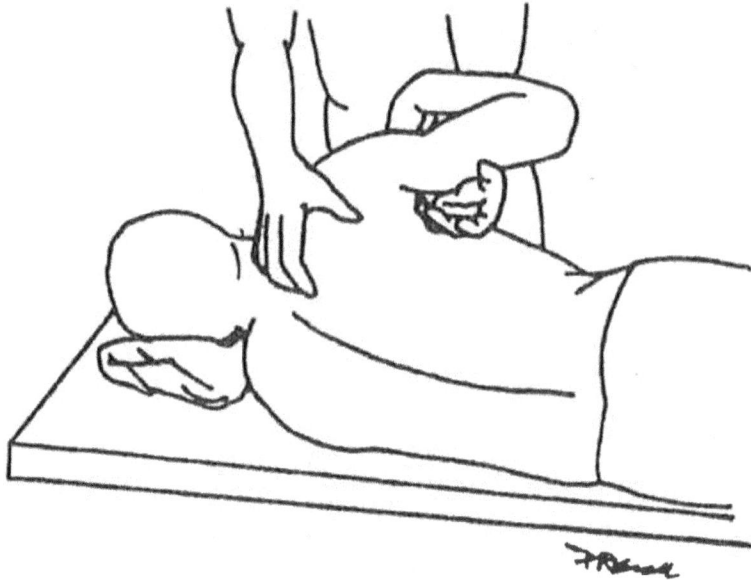

Figure 10. Sidelying treatment of upper extremity

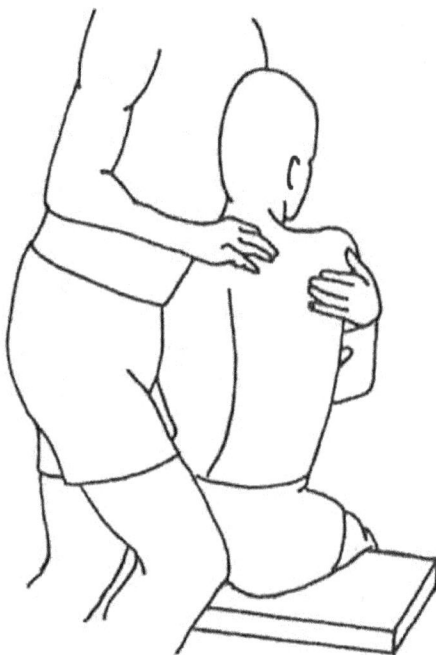

Figure lla. Seated inhalation treatment. Trunk

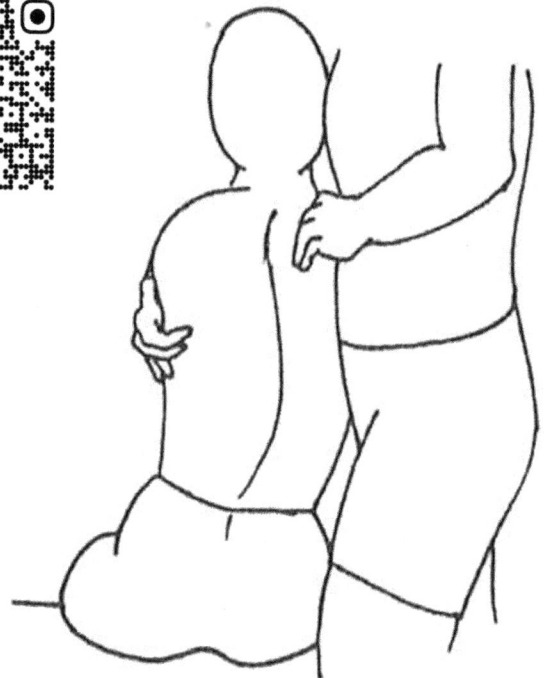

Figure llb. Seated exhalation treatment. Trunk

Functional Approach to the Thoracic Cage

Costal Cage Responses to Motion Testing

1. Exhalation Restriction

- Free Motions Introduced Through Upper Extremity

   Internal Rotation

   Adduction

   Caudad Traction*

- Free Motions Introduced Through Trunk

   Ipsilateral Rotation and Side-bending

   Extension (Backward Bending)

   Lateral Translation to Same Side

   Anterior Translation

   Cephalad Distraction*

2. Inhalation Restriction

- Free Motions Introduced Through Upper Extremity

   External Rotation

   Abduction

   Cephalad Compression*

- Free Motions Introduced Through Trunk

   Contralateral Rotation and Side-bending

   Flexion (Forward Bending)

   Lateral Translation to Same Side

   Posterior Translation

   Cephalad Distraction*

*May occasionally be opposite

Functional Approach to Thoracic Cage
Viscerosomatic Inputs·

- Viscerosomatic or somatovisceral reflex changes exhibit a linkage phenomenon between the lateral and midline columns. Motion responses palpated in either column exhibit identical response characteristics (See Figure 12.); however, side-bending introduced through the head and neck will exhibit mirror-image findings when compared to the side-bending response introduced through the thorax (lack of accord).

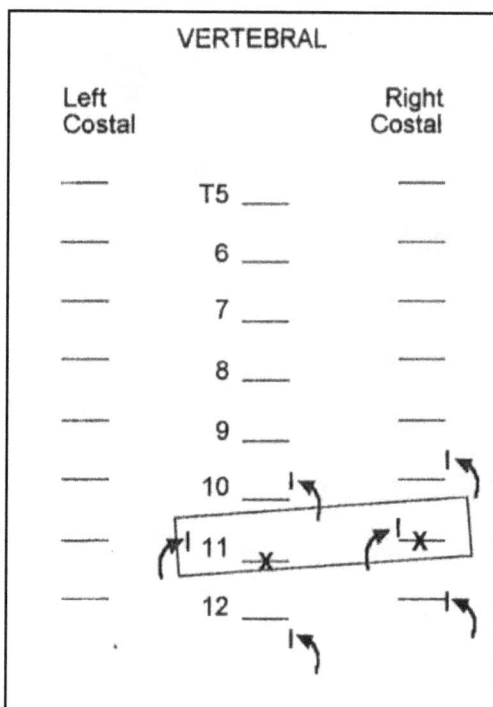

Figure 12.
Schematic representation of linkage at T-11 with right rib 11. Arrows at each indicate resistance to passive axial rotation to the right. Opposing symmetries are indicated for adjacent segments (superiorly and inferiorly) in each vertical column.

- Linkage phenomena is also associated with states of disequilibrium and shock from sympathetic nervous system activation.

-     Treatment can be carried out by introducing cervical and ipsilateral lower extremity motions responding with ease at the dysfunctional rib. While seated, test at the dysfunctional rib for motion responses to AP translation and head rotation. Position the patient according to the prone or supine (posterior or anterior translation) preference. Head rotation left or right is also positioned by the patient as they assume the prone or supine position. The operator stands on ipsilateral side introducing motions through the patient's lower extremity, which respond with ease at the dysfunctional rib (flexion/extension, abduction/adduction, internal/external rotation, cephalad/caudad translation, inhalation/exhalation).

Figure VI-2. Motion procedures applied through the leg, supine; the operator has the subject's right knee semi-flexed and fixed ·within the examiner's right axilla. This facilitates motion input through the lower extremity: cephalad/caudad, flexion/extension, inversion/eversion or abduction/ adduction.

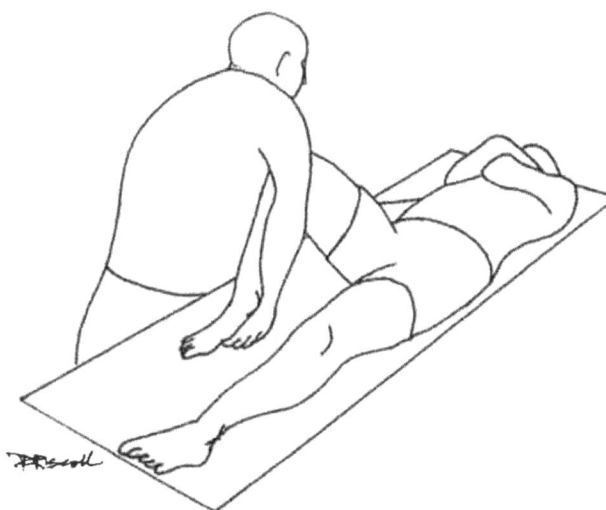

Figure VI-3. . Motion procedures applied through the leg, prone; the operator has the subject's right knee semi-flexed and fixed between the examiner's left arm and rib cage. The same element of control is gained by using the left hand to provide support at the knee.

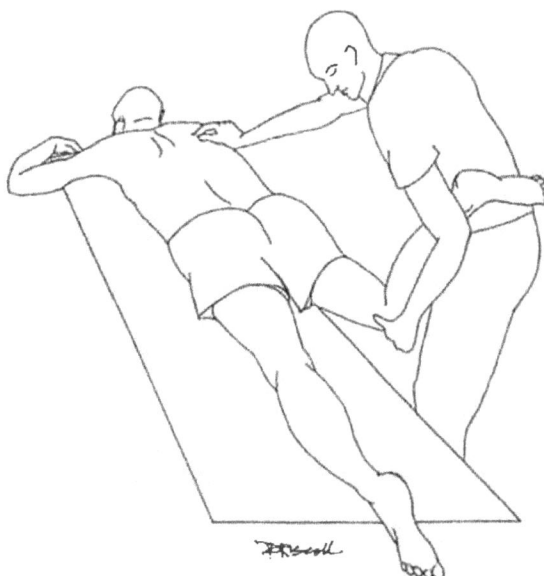

THORACIC CAGE DIAGNOSIS

LOCALIZE 3-SEGMENT COMPLEX USING PERCUSSION
AND MOTION

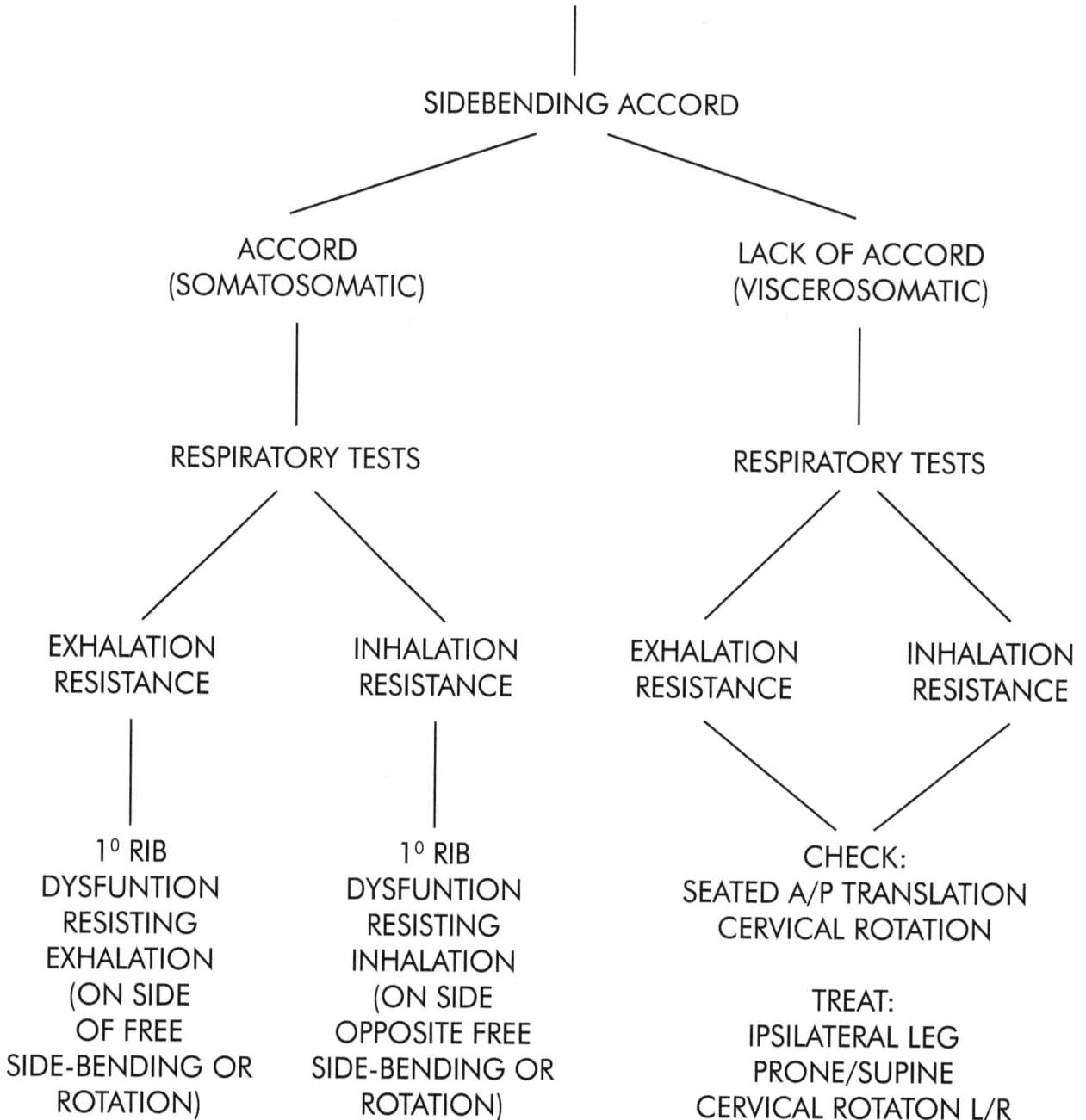

SIDEBENDING ACCORD

ACCORD
(SOMATOSOMATIC)

LACK OF ACCORD
(VISCEROSOMATIC)

RESPIRATORY TESTS

RESPIRATORY TESTS

EXHALATION
RESISTANCE

INHALATION
RESISTANCE

EXHALATION
RESISTANCE

INHALATION
RESISTANCE

1^0 RIB
DYSFUNTION
RESISTING
EXHALATION
(ON SIDE
OF FREE
SIDE-BENDING OR
ROTATION)

1^0 RIB
DYSFUNTION
RESISTING
INHALATION
(ON SIDE
OPPOSITE FREE
SIDE-BENDING OR
ROTATION)

CHECK:
SEATED A/P TRANSLATION
CERVICAL ROTATION

TREAT:
IPSILATERAL LEG
PRONE/SUPINE
CERVICAL ROTATON L/R

TREAT: IPSILATERAL UPPER EXTREMITY AND TRUNK

Motion Behavior

VERTEBRA	RESISTS SIDE-BENDING				RIB		RESISTS	
	shoulder/trunk		head/neck					
Location	to right?	to left?	to right?	to left?	right?	left?	inhal.?	exhal.?

Examiner: _____

Segmental Feedback Control and Afferent Reduction

The Concept of a Mobile Unit

The function of a mobile unit is to initiate and allow motion in a continuous smooth response to regional and whole-body demands. Dysfunction is reflected in tissues overlying segments through their ability to initiate, maintain, and allow for motion at that segment. Muscles have both an active and passive component, and function as the common final pathway in a neurologic system. Feedback is provided by proprioceptors and mechanoreceptors in all of the tissues surrounding the mobile unit. The resting tone of the muscle as well as qualities of the passive tissues, including fascial tension and tissue congestion, all influence the ability of the mobile unit to participate in coordinated motion.

The movement control system includes the articular surfaces between bony structures, the adnexal tissues (which move, allow movement, and stabilize position), and the CNS (which controls the moment to moment coordination of motion patterning, intensity and duration). Afferent input (feedback) is responsible for fine tuning this coordinated output along the final common neuro musculoskeletal (motor) pathway.

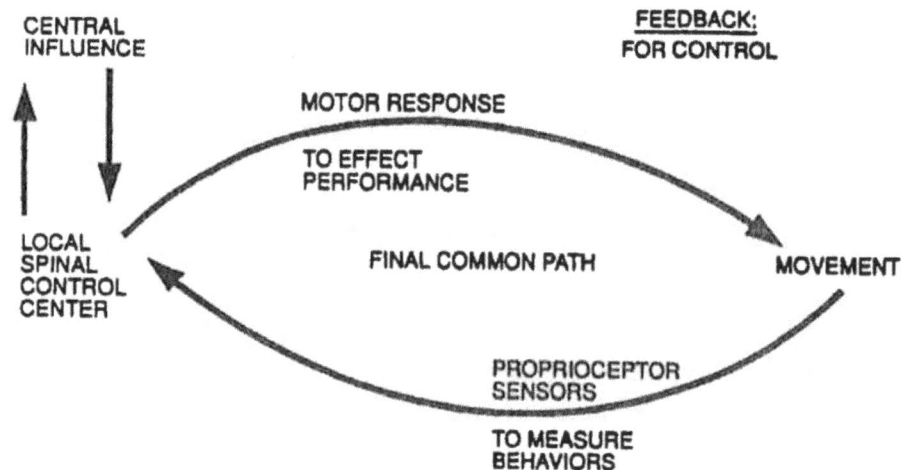

CENTRAL
INFLUENCE

FEEDBACK:
FOR CONTROL

MOTOR RESPONSE

TO EFFECT
PERFORMANCE

LOCAL
SPINAL
CONTROL
CENTER

FINAL COMMON PATH

MOVEMENT

PROPRIOCEPTOR
SENSORS

TO MEASURE
BEHAVIORS

Feedback control mechanisms help to maintain set points within operating systems. For example, the set point of a thermostat helps to keep the temperature constant, as well as an auto-pilot mechanism keeping the steering mechanism of an airplane on track. In this neuromuscular feedback system, afferent activity is a continuous response to gravity, balance, posture and movement in relation to force, position, velocity, and direction. The common final pathway of the neuromuscular control system functions to have all the parts in the right position at the right time to carry out postural and motion demands. The feedback system is primarily coming from the proprioceptors and mechanoreceptors in the joint capsule in the ligaments, tendons, muscles, and skin. Visceral efferent activity also responds to motion demands placed on the motor system through circulatory, metabolic and visceral homeostatic functions. Disturbances in sensory input (afferent pathways) impairs homeostatic functions which, in turn, disturbs motor performance and feedback.

Facilitation of the segmental response occurs in association with increased resting tone and associated asymmetrical responses to motion demands, with the part not being in the right place at the right time. Such disturbances cause increased afferent stimulation and efferent responses overreact to attempt to bring the situation under control. The goal of manipulative technique is to minimize the effort necessary and the energy used to maintain midline posture and coordinated responses to motion demands. By reducing afferent input, functional techniques assist the body's natural tendency to reduce the resting tone of the efferent fibers, thereby expending less energy. As the sensitivity of the muscle spindle is rehabilitated through afferent reduction, the efferent tone (gamma system) is allowed to function optimally. Continued destimulation of afferent pathways allows for a cascade of responses in the central control mechanism that also influence circulatory and metabolic function over the course of days to weeks following treatment. There is a tendency to experience increased pain immediately following resolution of motor system dysfunctions. This is possibly related to the increased sensitivity of the afferent system occurring immediately after treatment.

ANTERIOR COSTAL CAGE

Sternochondral elements function as 2 mobile columns of segmentally organized articulations. Like the sacrum, its segmental (midline) components are fused so motion occurs on either side at the corresponding sternochondral junctures. No distinct motion responses are palpated at costochondral junctions; in fact, costovertebral and sternochondral dysfunctions appear to be independent of one another. Neither carries with it findings reflected in, or by, the other. (Linkage being the exception, where the same costovertebral finding is carried all the way to the sternum)

Anterior costal cage motor responses may be palpated throughout the sternochondral expanse focusing at a central segment with mirror-image responses above and below. Motion disturbances may occur across both columns as a single finding (see below picture to left) or across just the right or left side with no finding on the other side. (see below picture to right) Trunk and head side-bending accord is usually lacking in the latter (unilateral dysfunction) and present in the former (bilateral dysfunction).

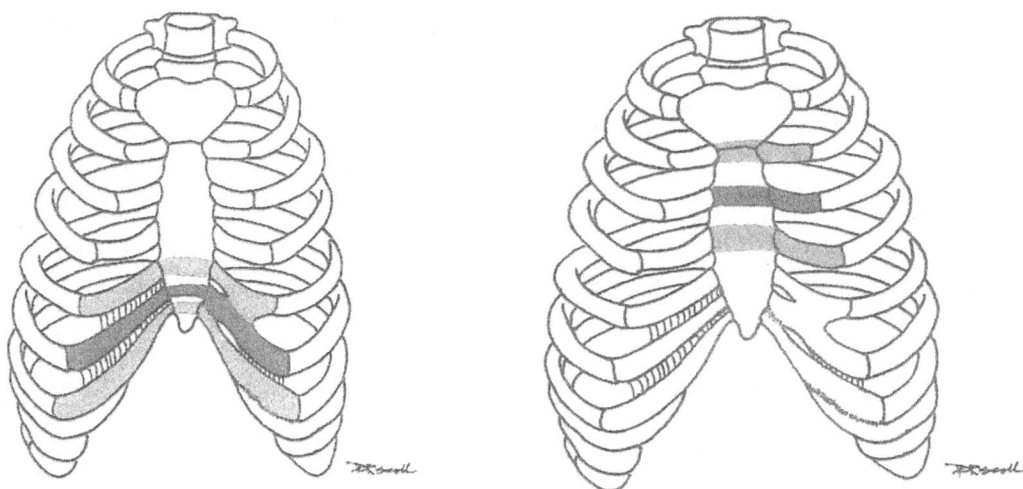

Scanning examination to locate sternochondral dysfunction begins supine, with simultaneous palpation of both sides of the sternum while introducing rotation from below through the legs. Repeated leg rotation is carried out while the operator's fingers move from segment to segment locating a central segment of dysfunction with mirror image findings above and below. The operator's attention is directed at whether the disturbance appears on both or just one side of the sternum and whether trunk and head side-bending responses are lacking accord.

Treatment is determined by testing responses of each leg individually, comparing motion towards and away from the midline, as well as flexion-extension and distraction compression of the hip. Directions of ease are combined in conjunction with head rotation, A/P translation of the shoulders and inhalation-exhalation to effect a resolution of the dysfunction palpated. (Upper extremity motions seem to carry no apparent association with sternochondral function).

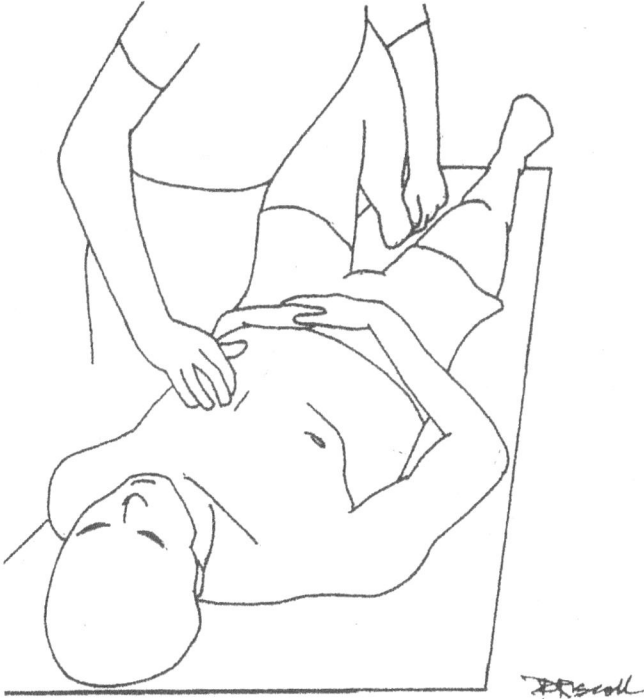

Treatment for Unilateral Sternochondral Dysfunction
(ipsilateral leg)

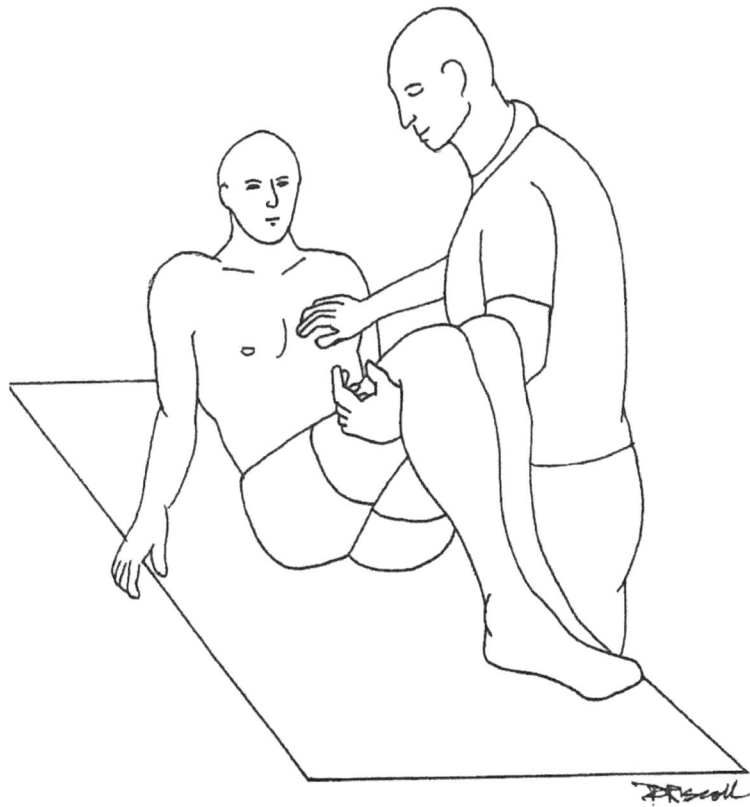

Treatment for Bilateral Sternochondral Dysfunction
- (legs together)

Functional Approach to the Sacropelvic Region

The sacropelvic area is considered as a whole and not as separate relationships between sacrum, ilium, and pubes. Mobile units are organized segmentally in five layers from S1 to S5, fanning out obliquely from the top of the sacrum to the femur. Sacropelvic dysfunctions can occur in one of two lateral columns, and are influenced by motions introduced through the extremities and the trunk.

Diagnostic Approaches to Sacropelvic Diagnosis

1. Standing percussion scan can localize the dysfunction in the midline column.
2. Side-lying tissue scan of medial ligamentous and lateral muscular tissues localizes the dysfunction to the left or right column. See Figures 2 and 3. Central, ligamentous, and muscular findings should be in an oblique line, consistent with a common segmental orientation. See Figure 4.

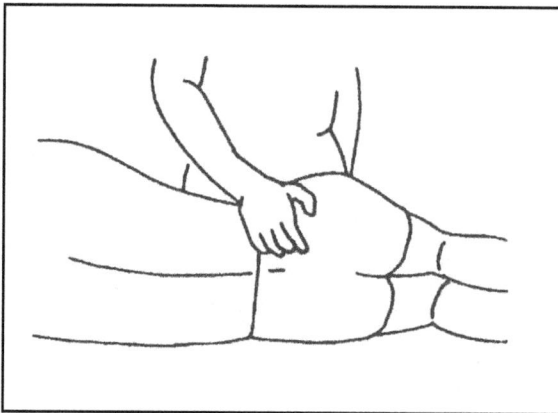

Figure 2. Subject is left sidelying for palpatory scan along the right sacroiliac ligamentous structure to determine location of any point(s) of increased tissue tension (resistance-to-pressure)

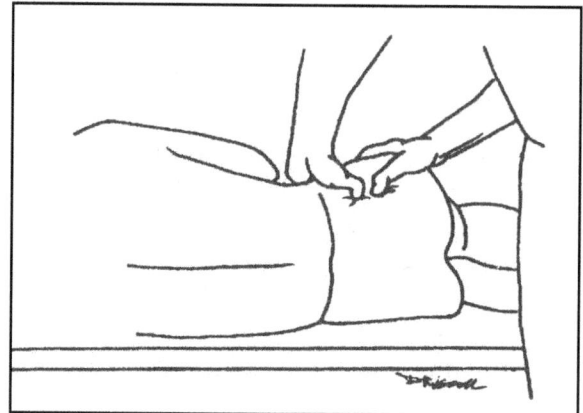

Figure 3. Subject is left sidelying for palpatory scan of right gluteal muscle mass. Examiner applies thumb pressure to determine location of any point(s) of increased muscle tension (resistance-to-pressure).

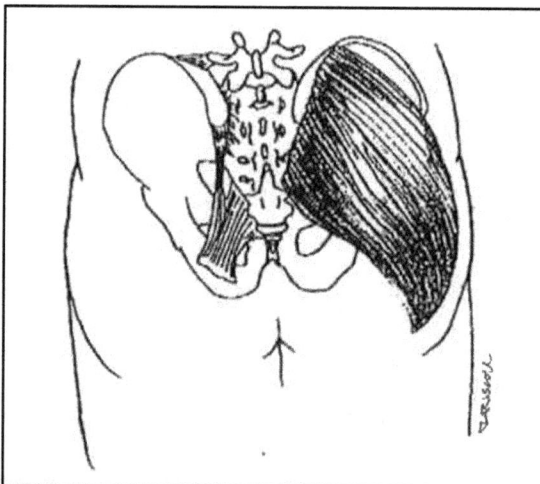

Figure 4. Diagrammatic illustration of lumbo-pelvic bony anatomic landmarks, functional sacroiliac ligaments (shown left), and right gluteal musculature.

3. Rotary scan supine to confirm the central segment and adjacent mirror-image findings. The use of the knees together introduces motion from below. See Figure 5.

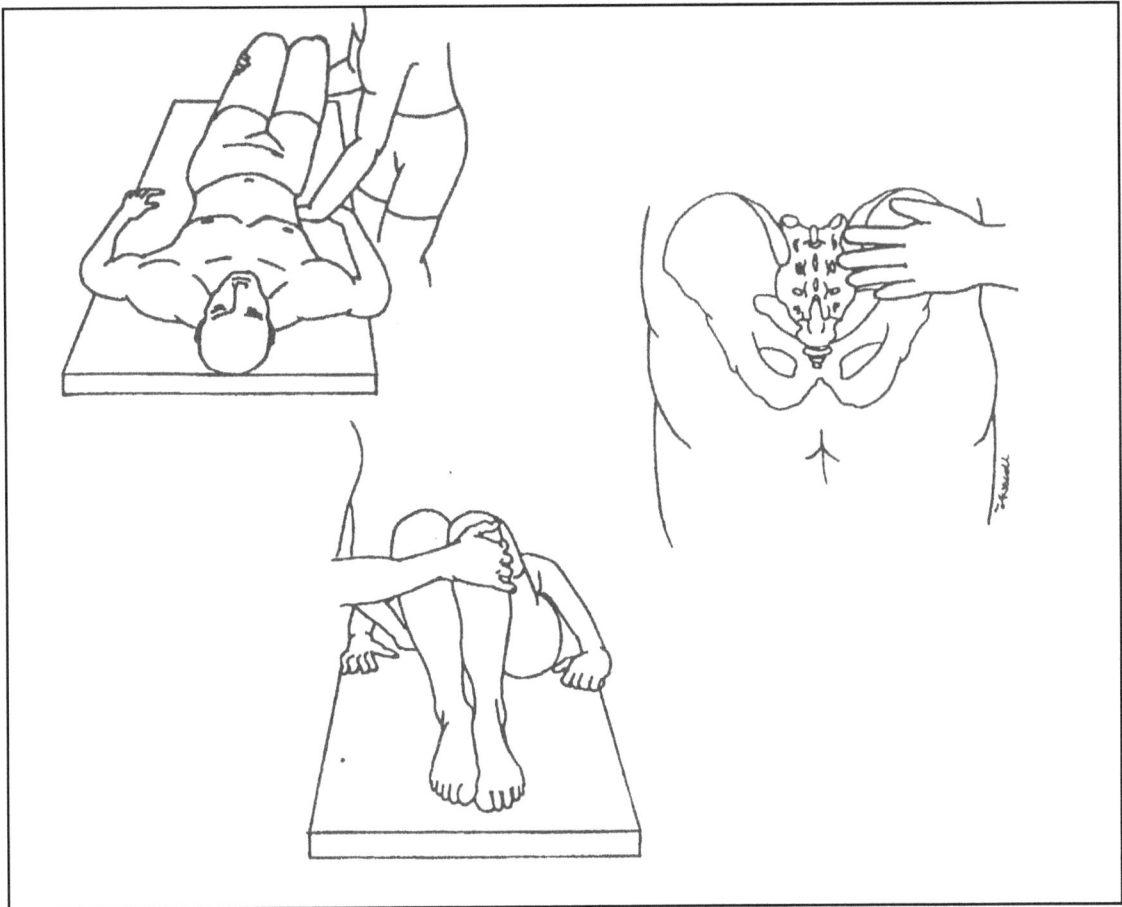

Figure 5. With the subject positioned supine, knees flexed and feet together resting on the table as a pivot point, the examiner scans throughout the lumbo-pelvic region using rotation to the right from below, introduced at the knees. Examiner's left fingertips monitor response at each lumbar spinous process and along the junction of the innominate to the sacro-coccygeal tip of the spine for local points lacking compliance to the rotary scan.

4. Rotary scan seated will confirm the supine findings, but will be introduced from the opposite side from above. See Figure 6

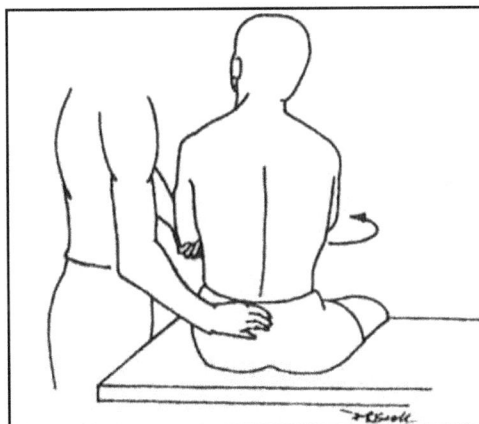

Figure 6.
Subject is seated for introduction of rotation left from above, controlled by the examiner's left hand grasp of the subject's arms folded, with response monitored by the right hand at spinal level S2.

Segmental Testing

5. Individual leg motions may be introduced supine in a medial and lateral direction. Responses to the initial introduction of these movements, not end range, reveal a characteristic pattern of responses in the sacropelvic region (see below) and functional treatment of these are combined with translatory and respiratory motions. See Figure 7.

Figure 7.
The examiner's right hand controls the right leg at the knee in motion medially to the left (shown) and then laterally to the right while the left hand monitors responses to compare compliance at a problem area identified at spinal level S2, right.

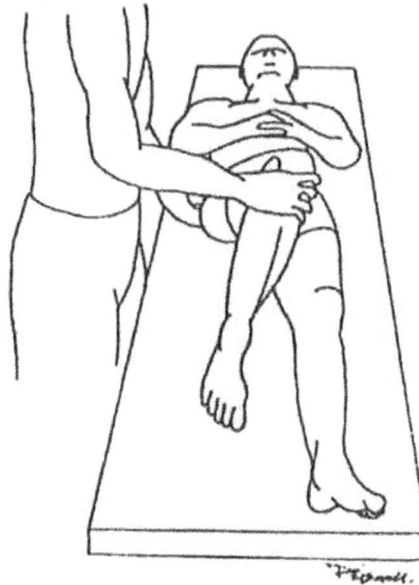

Retesting after treatment confirms that segmental responses of legs tested individually are resolved. If legs tested together are still asymmetrical, treatment through trunk or with legs together should be performed until findings resolve completely.

Pattern 1: Asymmetry with testing of the legs together as a unit. Individual leg testing reveals no asymmetrical responses. This is a midline column dysfunction, and can be treated using midline motions in either a seated or supine position.

Pattern 2: Asymmetry of the ipsilateral leg only. Treatment would be carried out using the ipsilateral leg in the direction of freedom, i.e., side-lying, with dysfunctional side up.

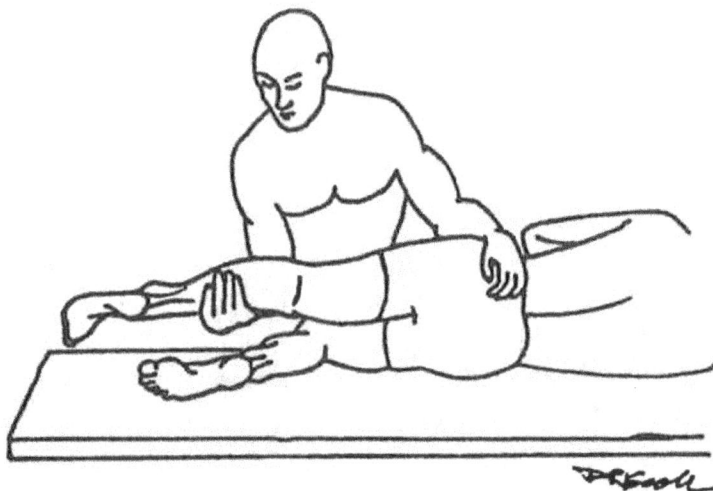

Pattern 3: Asymmetry of each leg individually.

- All but one leg direction restricted. (One free direction is found on contralateral leg.) Treat prone or supine using the one free leg to introduce motions responding with ease at the dysfunctional segment.

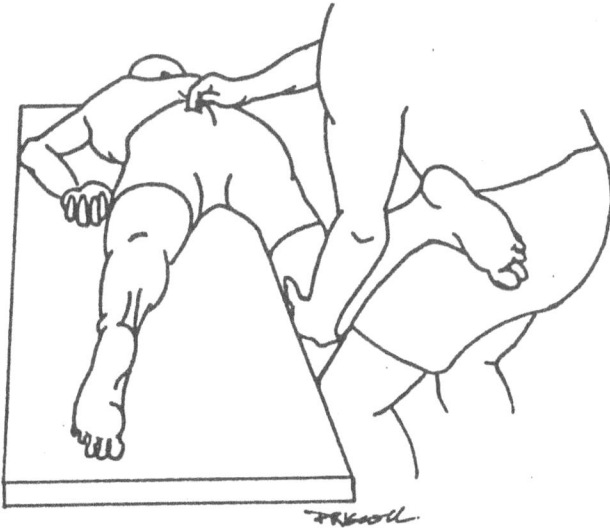

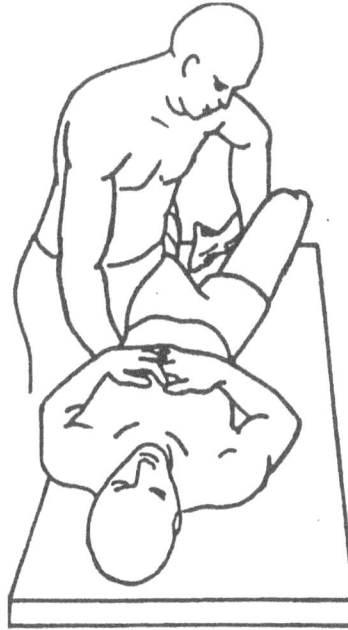

- Each leg with one free and one restricted direction.
    a) Restriction of each leg in the same directions, left or right. Treatment is supine with the legs together introducing directions responding with ease at the dysfunctional segments.

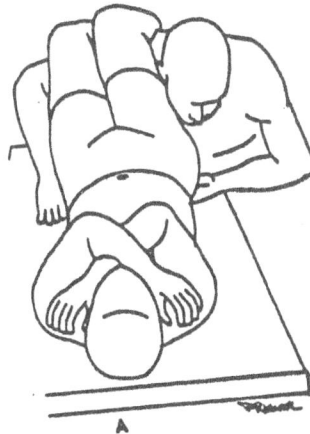

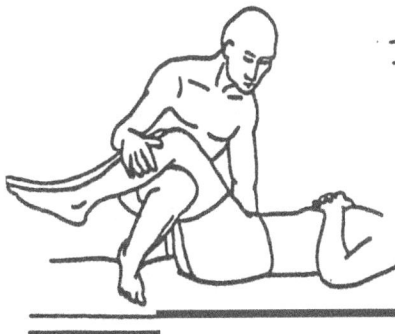

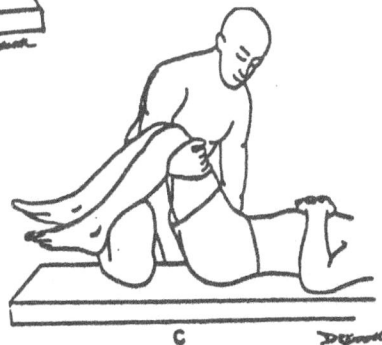

b) Restriction of each leg in the opposite directions, towards the midline or away from the midline treatment involves positioning the patient with legs crossed (free towards the midline) or ankles crossed with legs abducted and externally rotated (free away from the midline). Either way, the operator supports the legs on his/her thigh. Additional motions are introduced in the directions responding with ease. (more or less hip flexion, trunk side-bending and rotation, compression/distraction, inhalation/exhalation)

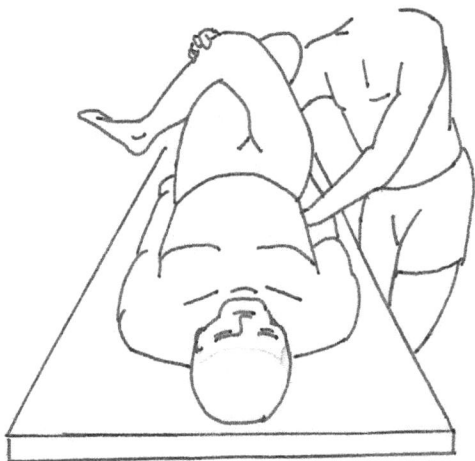

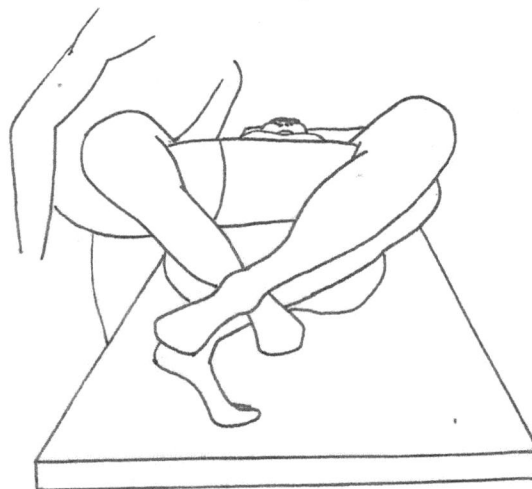

Treatment an also be carried out using a direct technique, in order to reduce the difficulty of managing the legs with indirect methods. In this case the legs are positioned in the direction that increases tension at the central segment in all directions. Muscle activation in the direction that increases tension can be used to enhance the response (squeezing the legs together against the operator's fist or pulling apart against the operator's counterforce)

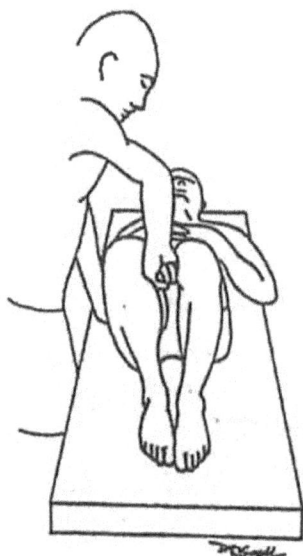

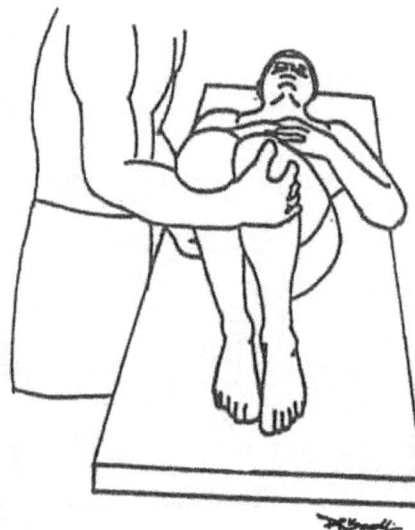

Motion Pattern Summary
SacroPelvis

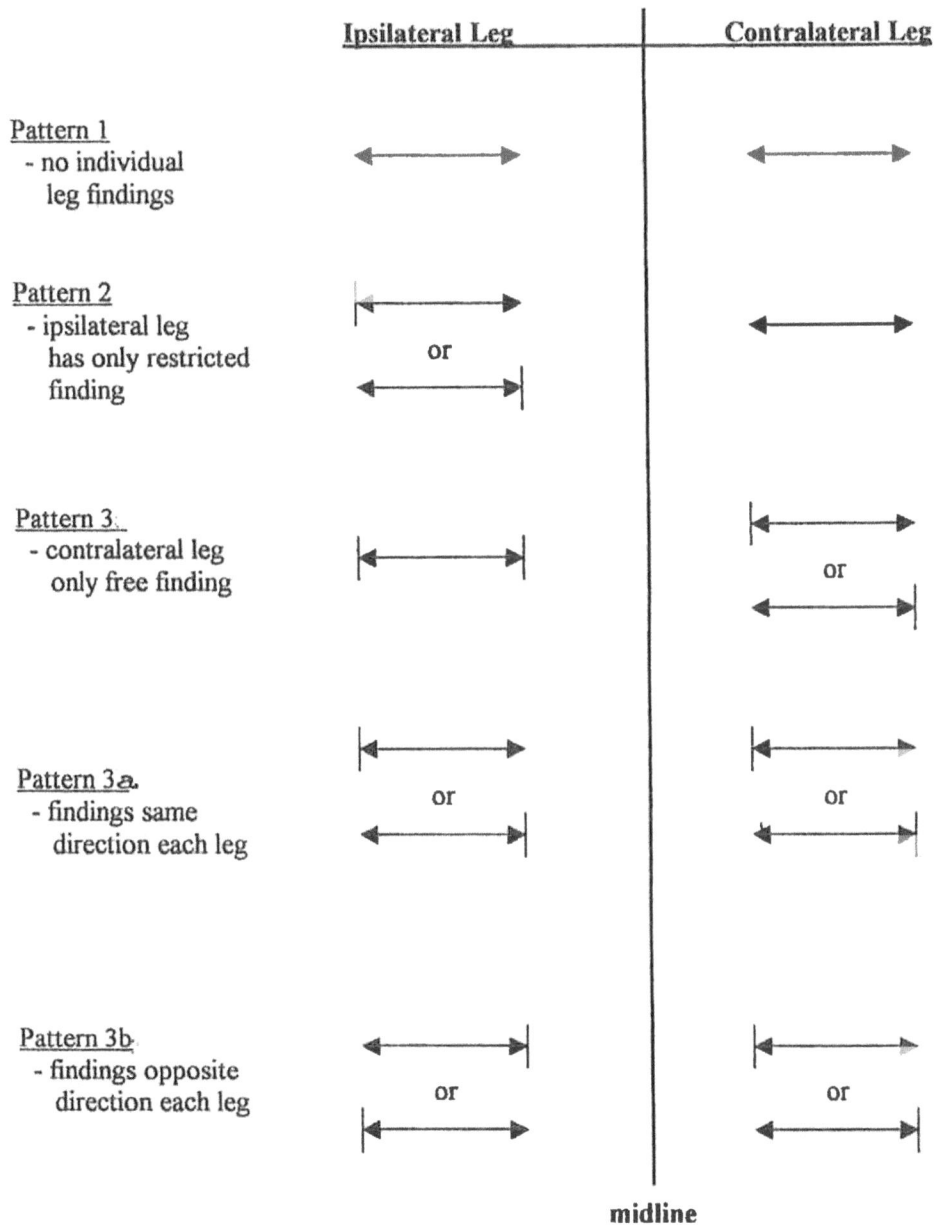

Ipsilateral Leg	Contralateral Leg

Pattern 1
- no individual
  leg findings

Pattern 2
- ipsilateral leg
  has only restricted
  finding

or

Pattern 3
- contralateral leg
  only free finding

or

Pattern 3a
- findings same
  direction each leg

or

Pattern 3b
- findings opposite
  direction each leg

or

midline

6. Areas of tissue tension in the lumbar and lower thoracic spine may be approached similarly due to the functional-relationship that may exist between these areas and the lower extremity. The same patterns found in the sacropelvis are applied.

Duplicate

Functional Approach to the Lower Extremities

LOWER EXTREMITY assessment and treatment similarly follows a regional sequence and interplay of functional relations between the thoracolumbar, lumbosacral and sacropelvic areas. Not only are lower extremity problems frequently resolved after treating these areas, but are as often used as levers to transmit the forces necessary to treat them successfully.

Functional motor programming in this region often follows coordinated patterns of motion and positioning of the lower extremity as a whole. These patterns may be used to enhance the effective response of tissue at a central segment anywhere in the appendage. Hip adduction/internal rotation is leveraged together with internal rotation of the tibia, knee flexion and plantar flexion/inversion of the ankle and forefoot (valgus). Similarly, hip abduction/external rotation can be used with external rotation of the tibia, knee flexion and dorsi-flexion/eversion of the ankle and forefoot (varus). Introducing a valgus or varus leverage is easily accomplished after testing motion responses at a particular central segment that favors one or the other. Fine-tuning is then carried out to position the entire extremity in a position that produces the greatest therapeutic response.

VALGUS

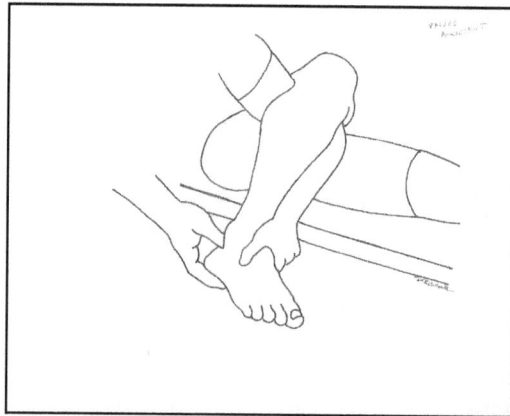

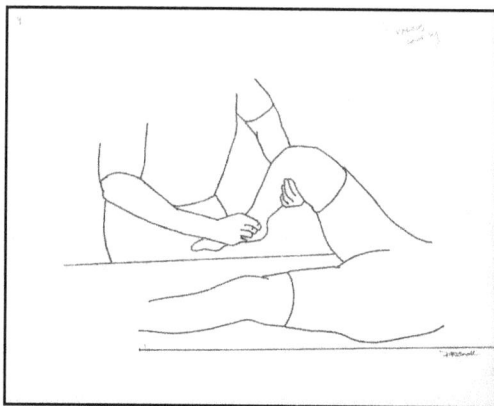
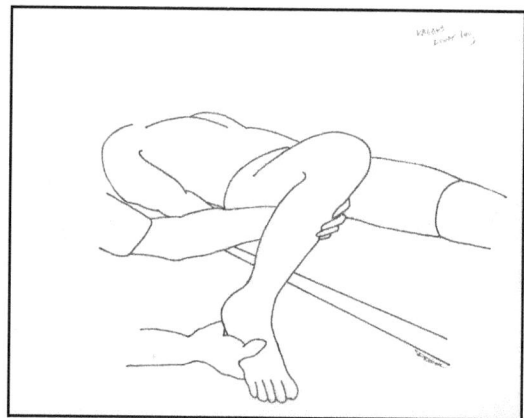

VARUS

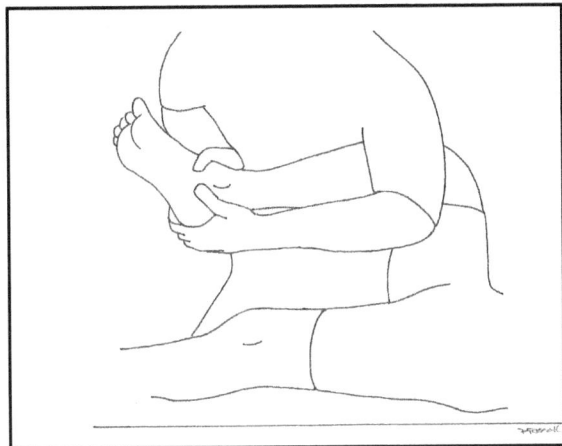 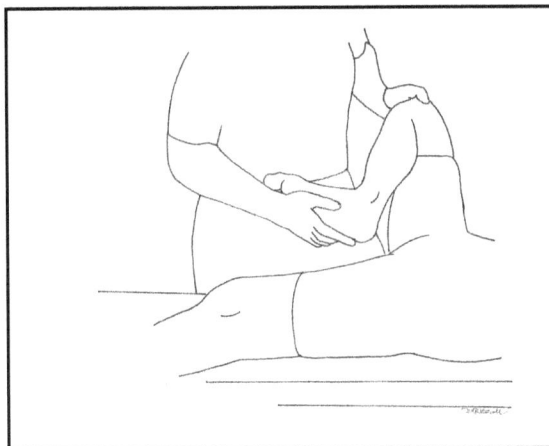

Diagnosis
1. Screen tissue (thigh/calf) for side of dysfunction using tissue resistance to pressure
2. Screen regional motion (hip/knee/ankle/foot)) to localize disturbed motion unit
3. Scan tissue segmentally to localize area of greatest tissue texture abnormality
4. Scan motion segmentally to identify central segment

Treatment
1. Test and position neighboring motion segments and the entire extremity optimizing responses of ease at the central segment.
2. Because of the larger size and lever action of extremity joints, greater forces and ranges of motion are often needed for optimal responses.
3. Treatment effectiveness is the result of optimizing responses to positioning of the entire extremity not from direct articulation of the local tissues.

Lower Extremity Motion Segments are not always shaped in a straight linear fashion but are often circular, semicircular or crescent shaped.
-Hip, medial and lateral
-Knee, tibio-femoral, fibulo-femoral, proximal tibio-fibular
-Ankle, talo-tibial, talo-fibular, distal tibio-fibular
-Foot, talus, calcaneus, navicular, cuboid, cuneiforms
-Toes

Functional Approach to the Upper Extremities

UPPER EXTREMITY diagnosis and treatment follows a natural sequence of functional interplay between neighboring regions, specifically between the craniocervical and cervicothoracic areas and the thoracic cage. Upper extremity problems often stem from disturbances in these areas, reflecting both neurological and mechanical sources of motor system imbalance. Conversely, upper extremity forces often play an important role in establishing and maintaining problems more centrally, as noted in the approach to costal cage treatment.

Generally, tissue dysfunction should be resolved centrally before evaluating and treating upper extremity problems. Once engaged, proximal and then distal extremity structures are assessed and treated, starting with the clavicle, which directly transmits and balances forces between midline and periphery.

A functional approach to the extremity focuses on a specific area of extremity motion disturbance identified using a single passive motion scan to locate the central segment of a three-part dysfunction, as we have done in the previous sections. Treatment is carried out by positioning neighboring motion segments and the extremity as a whole into relative positions of ease, palpated at the central segment.

Segmental testing has a neurologic basis for a three-segment relationship in the upper extremity based on the sensorimotor arrangement of dermatomes and myotomes. A central segment and its adjacent opposite segments can be palpated in response to passive motion testing anywhere in the body, including over muscles and ligaments!

Diagnosis
1. Screen tissue (arm/forearm) for side of dysfunction using tissue resistance to pressure
2. Screen regional motion (shoulder/forearm/wrist) to localize disturbed motion unit
3. Scan tissue segmentally to localize area of greatest tissue texture abnormality
4. Scan motion segmentally to identify central segment

Treatment
1. Test and position neighboring motion segments and the entire extremity optimizing responses of ease at the central segment.
2. Because of the larger size and lever action of extremity joints, greater forces and ranges of motion are often needed for optimal responses.
3. Treatment effectiveness is the result of optimizing responses to positioning of the entire extremity not from direct articulation of the local tissues.

Upper Extremity Motion Segments are not always shaped in a straight linear fashion but are often circular, semicircular or crescent shaped.
- **Clavicle**, sternal and acromial
- **Shoulder**, anterior, superior and posterior gleno-humeral
- **Elbow**, radio-ulnar, radio-humeral, medial and lateral ulno-humeral
- **Wrist**, radio-ulnar, carpo-radial, carpo-ulnar
- **Hand**, intercarpal, carpo-phalangeal
- **Fingers**

Unique Contributions of
William L. Johnston DO Functional Methods in
Osteopathic Manipulative Medicine

1. Determination of the presence of Somatic Dysfunction using a standardized screening exam that describes the tests and the criteria for eliciting positive findings on which to base the diagnosis of Somatic Dysfunction. Two tests each for motion, tissue and structure are applied to 8 regions of the body. Passive motion tests assess whether resistance to motion comes sooner in one direction versus the other without regard for end feel or end-range. Tissue findings are palpated as increased resistance to pressure. Somatic Dysfunction is determined regionally by the presence of at least one positive finding of motion or structure and one positive finding of tissue

2. Development and use of the percussion scan to localize specific segments of Somatic Dysfunction.

3. The use of scanning procedures (repetitive use of one test over many adjacent segments) to identify a three-segment complex where the central segment behaves exactly opposite to the adjacent segments above and below.

4. Discovery of unique thoracic cage relationships between the central spinal and lateral costal columns where the central segments of each are related functionally as either linked (motion responses the same across columns) or non-linked (motion responses the opposite across columns).

5. Discovery of an additional motion testing response using head side-bending accord to quickly determine if the relationship between the spinal and costal columns is non-linked (in accord) or linked (lacking accord).

6. Discovery of unique functional relationships between the extremities and costal cage dysfunctions that are used to resolve linked dysfunctions using the lower extremity, and non-linked dysfunctions using the upper extremity.

7. Development of motion tests to assess segmental motor system function in areas where bones are fused across multiple segments (i.e. sacrum and sternum).

8. Application of the three-segment mobile complex of localizing somatic dysfunction to the two mobile columns of the anterior costal cage (sterno chondral articulations) and to the sacro-pelvis (sacro-iliac articulations) and characterizing that dysfunction using individual leg motion responses.

Clinical Considerations

- Thoracic cage reflexes activate motor programs throughout the entire weight bearing system. These programs coordinate function between the 3 major body regions: head/neck, thorax and pelvis. Gross motion introduced in any one of these regions is coupled with relative motion in the opposite direction in the adjacent region. (Gait mechanics coordinate head, arm and leg swing all in opposite directions).

- Neighboring or distant regions may be used to enhance treatment responses anywhere in the body. (A/P relation of shoulders and pelvis) craniocervical positioning may enhance upper thoracic treatment (supine) mandible positioning may enhance upper cervical treatment (supine) ankle or metatarsal positioning may enhance costal treatment
  - A/P relation between shoulders and hips
  - Craniocervical positioning may enhance upper thoracic treatment responses
  - Head, face and mandible positioning may enhance cervical treatment responses
  - Ankle or metatarsal positioning may enhance thoracic cage and/or sacropelvic treatment responses
  - Eye movements and teeth clenching may enhance thoracic cage treatment responses

- Functional methods can be applied to areas of the body that are anatomically or surgically different than normal. Fused joints, for example, do not move but they do have segmental motor responses and so participate in movement nonetheless. Their response to motions introduced passively can be palpated and treated functionally. Likewise, for any joint or bony anomaly, known or unknown, that might impair or alter mobility or compromise the safety of a forceful manipulative intervention, motion responses that reflect its segmental function can be easily palpated and safely treated with Functional technique.

- Positioning the patient for optimal treatment response can be accomplished in almost any situation where the patient may be bedridden or can only lie pain-free in certain ways. Functional approaches can be modified and directions of ease accomplished in positioning the patient before introducing motion passively. For example, side-bending left accompanies right side-lying, while A/P translation, flexion/extension, and rotation are also easily positioned side-lying.

- Functional palpation skills take time to develop, but can be attuned not only to responses of the motor system, but as we have seen, to ligamentous and connective tissue responses as well. We know when disturbed tissues are treated with any manipulative technique fluid function is enhanced, as dysfunction is resolved. This fluid response is also palpable and can be appreciated when the operator holds the functional treatment position a bit longer. Therapeutic fluid responses in the entire body may also be mobilized with these approaches.

Appendix

Course Forms

Often during the course of teaching Functional Methods I have elected to do data collection on inter-examiner reliability to see if the tests learned and findings elicited have any reproducibility. One of our goals in teaching Functional Methods is to elevate the science of our practice by making the testing procedures as uniform as possible. That includes not only the description of how to perform the tests but also how to interpret them and record them in as uniform a manner as is possible. In order for what we do with our palpation skills to be considered objective the palpatory findings we observe must be reproducible. That means that the same findings are observed by multiple examiners performing the same tests on the same subjects.

In an effort to further the exploration of this essential aspect of clinical science and enhance our ability to establish that in fact our testing methods are objective, I have included some forms that will facilitate the documentation of verifying this objectivity. They include the three types of testing procedures that we employ; screening, scanning and segmental tests of the neuromusculoskeletal system, which have been addressed in this text.

The first form lists the 48 tests used in the screening exam dividing them into tests of structure, tissue and motion. Using this form, the examiner can record each finding and using the second form, Record of Screening Exam which is divided into regions, insert the test number of any and all positive findings. Regional Somatic Dysfunction can be easily determined by regions having a positive tissue finding and either a positive motion or structural finding. Examiners and subjects can be given numbers so that the forms reveal no ones identity and allow for easy comparison for multiple examiners performing the tests on the same subject.

Additionally, there is a final form that details the specific findings of segmental motion testing in the thoracic cage. (Record of Segmental Motion Behavior) The form can be used a number of ways but my preference is for the instructor to identify a 3 segment complex in the thoracic cage, noting and even marking on the subject with a colored dot the vertebral level of that dysfunction. Multiple levels can be identified with subsequent performance of the segmental tests listed by multiple examiners at that same vertebral level. Specific palpatory tests represented on the form include responses noted at the indicated vertebral level when side-bending is introduced through the trunk and the head, whether the rib dysfunction is to the right or left, and if that rib exhibits resistance to inhalation or exhalation.

The uniformity of the tests applied, the interpretation of the palpatory responses elicited and the manner in which the findings are recorded are the main factors influencing the success or failure of reproducibility and inter-examiner reliability. Please contact the author at drhfriedman@gmail.com with any feedback.

Registration Information

Name _____ Date of Birth _____

Address _____

Country _____ Country Code _____

Phone _____ Email _____ Sex _____

School Attended _____

Functional Classes Taken: _____

_____

_____

_____

Private Practice   Yes   No   Location _____

Teaching Faculty   Yes   No   School _____

Student   Yes   No   School _____

Other _____

Medical Problems List: _____

_____

_____

Surgical History: _____

_____

_____

Class Participation Number _____

RECORD OF SCREENING TESTS TO CHARACTERIZE REGIONAL SOMATIC DYSFUNCTION

Structure	1	Inferior mastoid process	L	R	
	2	Inferior first rib at anterior trap	L	R	
	3	Inferior acromion	L	R	
	4	Inferior scrapular angle	L	R	
	5	Inferior iliac crest	L	R	
	6	Inferior trochanter	L	R	
	7	Inferior plantar arch	L	R	
	8	Lumbar convexity	L	R	
	9	Costal cage rotation	L	R	
	10	Anterior pelvis	L	R	
	11	Anterior sholder	L	R	
	12	Anterior orbit	L	R	
	13	Jaw deviation - relaxed, open	L	R	
	14	Cervical lordosis	I	D	N (increased, decreased, normal)
	15	Thoracic kyphosis	I	D	N
	16	Lumbar lordosis	I	D	N
Tissue	17	Calf tissue tension	L	R	
	18	Thigh tissue tension	L	R	
	19	Gluteal tissue tension	L	R	
	20	Sacral tissue tension increased?	Y	N	
	21	Lower lumbar tissue tension increased?	Y	N	
	22	Upper lumbar tissue tension increased?	Y	N	
	23	Lower thoracic tissue tension increased?	Y	N	
	24	Upper thoracic tissue tension increased ?	Y	N	
	25	Lower cervical tissue tension increased?	Y	N	
	26	Upper cervical tissue tension increased?	Y	N	
	27	Jaw muscle tension - relaxed	L	R	
	28	Jaw muscle tension - clenched	L	R	
	29	Forearm tissue tension	L	R	
	30	Upper arm tissue tension	L	R	
	31	Upper anterior costal cage tissue tension	L	R	
	32	Lower lateral costal cage tissue tension	L	R	

Motion resistance encountered at the initiation of passive

	33	Hyperextension of knees	L	R	
	34	Lateral shift of pelvis	L	R	
	35	One leg standing (stork) test	L	R	
	36	Restricted active lumbar side - bending	L	R	
	37	Does rotation occur into concavity in 36?	Y	N	
(seated)	38	Forearm pronation	L	R	
	39	Shoulder/trunk side - bending	L	R	
	40	Shoulder/trunk rotation	L	R	
	41	Head/neck side - bending	L	R	
	42	Head/neck rotation	L	R	
(supine)	43	Lateral leg swing	L	R	
	44	Upper anterior costal cage inhalation	L	R	
	45	Lower lateral costal cage inhalation	L	R	
	46	Arms abducted overhead	L	R	
	47	CRI vault hold	H	W	N (hyperactive, weak, normal)
	48	Restriction of flexion or extension?	Y	N	

Record of Regional Screening Exam

	Altered			Somatic Dysfuntion
	Tissue Texture	Motion	Structure	
Head/Face				
Cervical				
Thoracic				
Lumbar				
Sacro-pelvic				
Costal Cage				
Upper Exrem				
Lower Extrem				

Subject: _____

Examiner: _____

	Altered		
	Tissue Texture	Motion	Structure
Head/Face	27 28	47 48	12 13
Cervical	25 26	41 42	1 14
Thoracic	23 24	39 40	3 15
Lumbar	21 22	36 37	8 16
Sacro-pelvic	19 20	34 35	5 10
Costal Cage	31 32	44 45	2 9
Upper Exrem	29 30	38 46	4 11
Lower Extrem	17 18	33 43	6 7

* Standardized for six tests per region: two tissue, two motion, two structure.

* **Criteria for regional somatic dysfunction:**
  one positive tissue test and
  one positive motion or structure test in any one region

Record of Regional Screening Exam

	Altered			Somatic Dysfuntion
	Tissue Texture	Motion	Structure	
Head/Face				
Cervical				
Thoracic				
Lumbar				
Sacro-pelvic				
Costal Cage				
Upper Exrem				
Lower Extrem				

Subject: _____

Examiner: _____

	Altered		
	Tissue Texture	Motion	Structure
Head/Face	27 28	47 48	12 13
Cervical	25 26	41 42	1 14
Thoracic	23 24	39 40	3 15
Lumbar	21 22	36 37	8 16
Sacro-pelvic	19 20	34 35	5 10
Costal Cage	31 32	44 45	2 9
Upper Exrem	29 30	38 46	4 11
Lower Extrem	17 18	33 43	6 7

* Standardized for six tests per region: two tissue, two motion, two structure.

* **Criteria for regional somatic dysfunction:**
  one positive tissue test and
  one positive motion or structure test in any one region

Record of Segmental Motion Behavior

Vertebra	Resists Side-Bending				Rib		Resists	
Location	Shoulder/Trunk		Head/Neck					
Location	to right?	to left?	to right?	to left?	to right?	to left?	inhal.?	exhal.?

Subject: _____

Examiner: _____

Record of Segmental Motion Behavior

Vertebra	Resists Side-Bending				Rib		Resists	
Location	Shoulder/Trunk		Head/Neck					
Location	to right?	to left?	to right?	to left?	to right?	to left?	inhal.?	exhal.?

Subject: _____

Examiner: _____

Course Schedule

Functional Methods - Part I

DAY 1

800 am	*(0900)*	Functional Methods—Conceptual Development
830 am	*(0930)*	Introduction to Functional Problem-Solving
915 am	*(1015)*	Selection of Regional Tests: Demonstration of Screening Exam
945 am	*(1045)*	Break/Clinical Exhibits
1000 am	*(1100)*	Screening Exam Demonstration (continued)
1100 am	*(1200)*	Percussion Scan: Spinal Regions
1145 am	*(1245)*	Lunch
100 pm	*(1400)*	Scanning Exam to Localize Dysfunctional Behavioral Motor Complex

- Respiratory Localization

- Side-Bending Localization

145 pm	*(1445)*	Introduction to Diagnosis and Treatment of Segmental Motion Dysfunction
215 pm	*(1515)*	Cervical Spine- Demonstration and Practice

- Segmental Motion Testing and Functional Manipulation

300 pm	*(1600)*	Break/Clinical Exhibits
315 pm	*(1615)*	Cervical Spine (continued)
400 pm	*(1700)*	Thoracic Spine – Demonstration and Practice

- Segmental Motion Testing and Functional Manipulation of:

  - mid-thoracic spine (using trunk)

  - upper-thoracic spine (using head)

  - lower-thoracic spine (using legs)

500 pm	*(1800)*	Adjourn

Course Schedule
Functional Methods - Part 1

DAY 2

800 am	*(0900)*	Thoracic Spine (continued)
900 am	*(1000)*	Segmental Feedback Control and Affected Reduction
945 am	*(1045)*	Break/Clinical Exhibits
1000 am	*(1100)*	Functional Approach to the Thoracic Cage
1045 am	*(1145)*	Thoracic Cage – Demonstration and Practice
		• Segmental Motion Testing for Rib Dysfunction
1145 am	*(1245)*	Lunch
100 pm	*(1400)*	Thoracic Cage – Demonstration and Practice
		• Functional Manipulation of Ribs Resisting Exhalation and Inhalation
245 pm	*(1545)*	Break/Clinical Exhibits
300 pm	*(1600)*	Thoracic Cage – Demonstration and Practice
		• Diagnosis and Treatment of Costovertebral Linkage
500 pm	*(1800)*	Adjourn

Course Schedule
Functional Methods - Part 1

DAY 3

800 am (*0900*)   Thoracic Cage (continued)

945 am (*1045*)   Break/Clinical Exhibits

1000 am (*1100*)   Anterior costal Cage

           • Sternochondral Responses to Somatic and Visceral Inputs

1045 am (*1145*)   Anterior Costal Cage – Demonstration and Practice

           • Functional Manipulation of Sternochondral Dysfunction

1230 pm (*1330*)   Adjourn

Course Schedule
Functional Methods - Part 2

DAY 1

800 am (*0900*)   Course Introduction

830 am (*0930*)   Thoracic Cage - Review

945 am (*1045*)   Break/Clinical Exhibits

1000 am (*1100*) Thoracic Cage – Review

1145 am (*1245*) Lunch

100 pm (*1400*)   Cervical spine – Review

245 pm (*1545*)   Break

300 pm (*1600*)   Upper Extremity – Demonstration and Practice

                  • Segmental Motion Testing and Functional Manipulation

500 pm (*1800*)   Adjourn

Course Schedule

Functional Methods - Part 2

DAY 2

800 am (*0900*)   Upper Extremity – Continued

945 am (*1045*)   Break

1000 am (*1100*) Sacropelvis – Demonstration and Practice

                    • Segmental Motion Testing

1145 am (*1245*) Lunch

100 pm (*1400*)   Sacropelvis – Demonstration and Practice

                    • Segmental Motion Testing and Functional Manipulation

245 pm (*1545*)   Break

300 pm (*1600*)   Lumbar Spine – Demonstration and Practice

                    • Segmental Motion Testing and Functional Manipulation

500 pm (*1800*)   Adjourn

Course Schedule
Functional Methods - Part 2

DAY 3

800 am (*0900*)   Review

830 am (*0930*)   Lower Extremity – Demonstration and Practice

  • Segmental Motion Testing and Functional Manipulation

945 am (*1045*)   Break

1000 am (*1100*) Lower Extremity – Demonstration and Practice

  • Segmental Motion Testing and Functional Manipulation

1145 am (*1245*) Clinical Integration

100 pm (*1400*)   Adjourn

About the Author...

Dr. Friedman, a fellow of the American Academy of Osteopathy, is a world renowned Osteopathic specialist who employs a multi-disciplinary approach to pain management and integrative wellness medicine. His practice incorporates Osteopathic Manipulative Medicine to diagnose and treat health problems of all types; musculoskeletal, neurologic, vascular, digestive, cardio-pulmonary, genitourinary and infectious. Osteopathic manipulation incorporates highly specialized palpatory skills to assess and treat disturbances in physiology and stimulate the health and vitality living within the patient.

Dr Friedman applies many types of manipulative approaches including Functional, Myofascial, Cranial, Viseral, Counterstrain, Muscle Energy, High Velocity/Low amplitude and Articulatory. He also uses therapeutic exercise, proprioceptive retraining, postural correction and various types of injections and works closely with other professionals providing Physical Therapy, Homeopathy, Chinese Medicine, Nutrition, Biofeedback and Psychotherapy.

Dr Friedman teaches internationally and has helped to establish Osteopathic programs around the world. He is co-founder of San Francisco International Manual Medicine Society and has written numerous books including Functional Methods, and a set of 3 instructional manuals in Counterstrain Approaches, Myofascial and Fascial Ligamentous Approaches and Primary Respiratory Mechanism Approaches. (www.sfimms.com) Dr Friedman has contributed chapters to numerous textbooks, conducts clinical research and has published articles in multiple journals.

Dr Friedman is in private practice in San Jose, California, he enjoys painting and Jazz music.

NOTES

NOTES

NOTES

SFIMMS SERIES IN NEUROMUSCULOSKELETAL MEDICINE

AUTHORS: Harry Friedman D.O., Wolfgang Gilliar D.O., Jerel Glassman D.O.

Osteopathic approaches to patient care offer the practitioner a variety of problem-solving and treatment options. Palpatory skill development establishes a basis for diagnostic assessment of neuromusculoskeletal function and its integrative role in maintaining health and overcoming disease. Osteopathic treatment and problem-solving skills apply a holistic approach that considers the therapeutic response of the whole patient. A variety of diagnostic and treatment methods have been developed to maximize outcomes.

This series of Osteopathic manipulative medicine texts presents a comprehensive course of instruction, including theory, palpation, diagnosis, and treatment. The thoughtful student will appreciate the detail and clarity of topic presentation and the sequence of skills development. Quality close-up photographic visuals accurately depict the table sessions using human and anatomic models.

COUNTERSTRAIN APPROACHES IN OSTEOPATHIC MANIPULATIVE MEDICINE

* Basic and intermediate level instructional manual
* Theoretical principles of indirect technique and spontaneous release by positioning
* Diagnostic application of tender point palpation for each body region
* Multiple therapeutic procedures presented for each tender point

MYOFASCIAL AND FASCIAL-LIGAMENTOUS APPROACHES IN OSTEOPATHIC MANIPULATIVE MEDICINE

* Basic and advanced level instructional manual
* Detailed connective tissue anatomy and physiology
* Theoretical principles of myofascial and fascial-ligamentous release
* Diagnostic and treatment approaches for each body region, including a myofascial screening exam
* Release enhancing maneuvers and multiple operator techniques
* Includes approaches of Dr.'s Ward, Chila, Becker, Barral and Sutherland

OSTEOPATHIC MANIPULATIVE MEDICINE APPROACHES TO THE PRIMARY RESPIRATORY MECHANISM

* Basic, intermediate, and advanced level instructional manual
* Anatomic relations and physiologic principles underlying the cranial concept
* Palpation exercises designed to facilitate diagnostic touch throughout the body
* Diagnostic and treatment approaches focus on fluid, membranous (dural), muscular, articular and bony aspects of the cranial mechanism, including a cranial screening exam
* Includes multiple operator techniques and approaches to infants and children

FUNCTIONAL METHODS IN OSTEOPATHIC MANIPULATIVE MEDICINE

* Presents Functional Methods approach developed by William L Johnston DO FAAO
* 2 basic level courses to cover all body regions
* Presents a unique palpation based understanding of the functional relationships between all body regions
* Diagnostic principles based on passive motion testing
* Treatment elegantly applies palpation based findings to restore proper relationships between body regions

email: admin@sfimms.com
www.sfimms.com

www.ingramcontent.com/pod-product-compliance
Lightning Source LLC
Chambersburg PA
CBHW061821210326
41599CB00034B/7075